Introduction

I've wanted to write a first aid book for years. As a Professional First Aid Trainer, I've used many books to assist my learners to understand and retain the knowledge necessary to become safe, prompt and effective first aiders. But I always felt the books I'd used, just lacked that personal touch. I wanted the books to explain the subjects to my learners in a way that was clear, straightforward, simple to understand and jargon free. A book that spoke to the learners in the same way I would, when actually stood up in a class teaching first aid.

I've tried to do all of these things when this writing this First Aid manual and the others in the series (CPR/AED & Paediatric First Aid). I hope that you feel that I am talking to you as an individual as you turn the pages of this book.

If you are reading this book because you are on a workplace First Aid course then you will see each chapter follows the learning outcomes and assessment criteria of both the TQUK Level 2 Award in Emergency First Aid at Work (QCF) and the TQUK Level 3 Award in First Aid at Work (QCF).

Since I wrote this book a few years ago, there have been many changes to the way first aid training is delivered, which have been outlined by the Health & Safety Executive (HSE), the Resuscitation Council (UK) and the European Resuscitation Council (ERC). This book has been updated in line with all of these recommendations.

This book complements the hands-on practical training you will receive from your first aid trainer and supports the underpinning knowledge necessary to be a competent and confident first aider.

And don't forget that first aid can be a life-saving skill and you never know when you may need to use it. Remember to keep this book safe and read it from time to time to keep your skills fresh.

I hope you enjoy my book and your first aid course.

David Howarth
Author

Disclaimer

The information contained in this book is for general information purposes only. The information is provided by the author and his agents and while we endeavour to keep the information up to date and correct, we make no representations or warranties of any kind, express or implied, about the completeness, accuracy, reliability, suitability or availability with respect to the book or the information, products, services, or related graphics contained in the book for any purpose. Any reliance you place on such information is therefore strictly at your own risk and the author highly recommends readers attend an instructor-led first aid training course provided by a suitably accredited first aid training provider. In no event will the author or his agents be liable for any loss or damage including without limitation, indirect or consequential loss or damage, or any loss or damage whatsoever arising from, or in connection with, the use of this book.

Contents

Roles & Responsibilities

2.1 What is a First Aider?

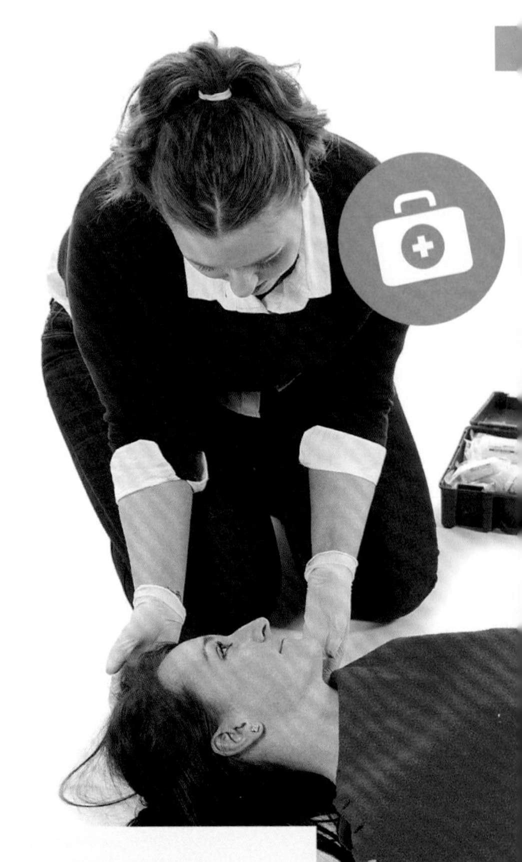

A first aider is someone who has attended a first aid course and is able to help someone else who has been injured or taken ill before the arrival of medical professionals like paramedics, doctors or nurses.

The aim of first aid is to make the casualty safe and comfortable, to treat any conditions they may have and of course... To make sure the casualty doesn't get any worse. Always ask the casualty (if responsive) for consent before touching them to administer first aid. This may help to reassure them and put them at ease.

2.2 Infection Control

As a first aider it is imperative that you protect yourself (and the casualty) from the risk of infection. Infections may come from germs or viruses contained on the skin or in body fluids, like blood and saliva.

Wearing simple equipment found in your first aid kit such as a face shield, plastic apron or disposable gloves can prove sufficient protection for you and the casualty.

Washing your hands properly prior to and immediately after treating a casualty will help reduce the risk of cross infection considerably. Dispose of waste in a clinical waste system.

2.3 Accident Reporting

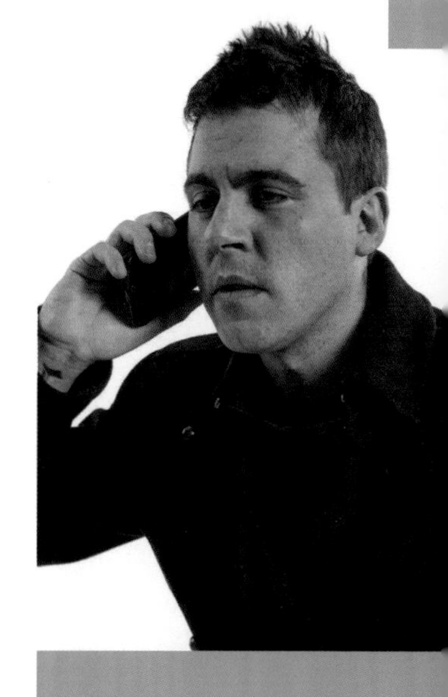

If the casualty's condition is serious you will need to call for help. Immediately dial 999/112 and ask for an ambulance. Send a bystander to do this or do this yourself by activating the speaker function of your mobile phone. Only leave the casualty alone if there is no other alternative. Be sure to tell them your name, if you are a first aider, to tell them how many casualties you have, what is wrong with the casualty(s), your exact location, and ensure the person making the call comes back to you to let you know what the ambulance service said.

After the arrival of the emergency services, tell them everything you know. If you are at work you will then be expected to complete an accident/incident report form.

Typically the form asks for:

- Details of the injured person
- Your information as the report writer
- When and where the accident happened
- What injuries or conditions were suffered?

'Immediately dial 999/112 and ask for an ambulance'

As a workplace first aider speak to your manager to learn what your company expects from you.

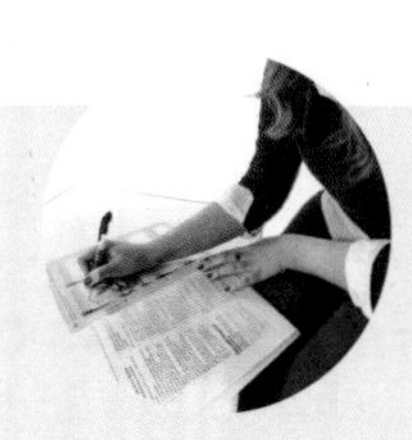

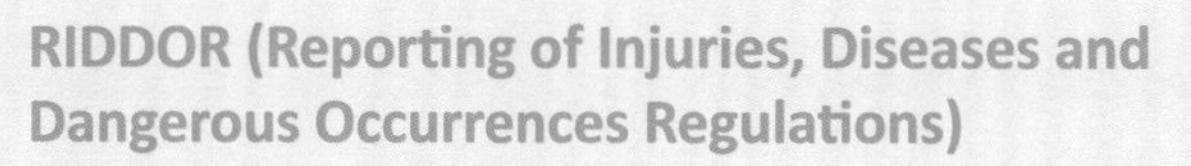

RIDDOR (Reporting of Injuries, Diseases and Dangerous Occurrences Regulations)

Accidents of a serious nature at work should be reported directly to the HSE. These incidents would include a death, major injury or over seven day injuries (these are injuries at work which cause the injured worker to be absent from work for more than seven days). Visit the HSE website for further details. www.hse.org.uk

2.4 First Aid Equipment

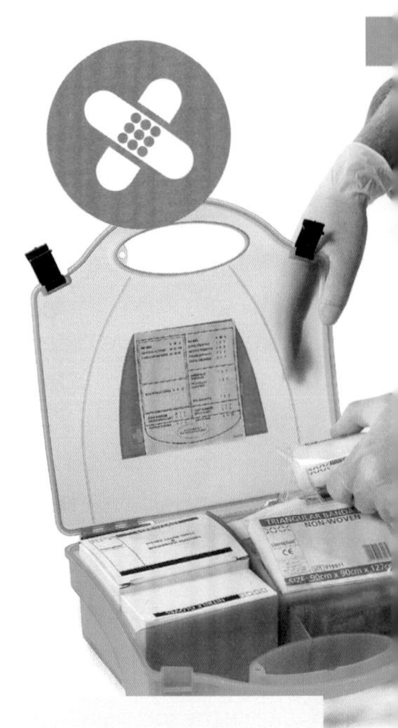

BS-8599-1 is the British Standard for first aid kits in the workplace.

These kits are available in different sizes to meet the needs of different sized companies (small, medium, large and travel).

To use first aid equipment safely, always:

- Use appropriate personal protective equipment (PPE)
- Always check bandages/dressings are within date
- Discard any items which may have been previously opened

For guidance here is a table of BS8599-1 compliant First Aid Kit contents:

CONTENTS	SMALL	MEDIUM	LARGE
Burn Relief Dressing 10cm x 10cm	1	2	2
Washproof Assorted Plasters	40	60	100
Large Dressing 18cm x 18cm Sterile	1	2	2
Medium Dressing 12cm x 12cm Sterile	4	6	8
Nitrile Gloves Pair	6	9	12
Mouth to Mouth Resuscitation Device	1	1	2
Finger Dressing with Adhesive Fixing 3.5cm	2	3	4
Conforming Bandage 7.5cm x 4m	1	2	2
Moist Cleansing Wipes	20	30	40
Single Use Triangular Bandage 90cm x 127cm	2	3	4
Universal Shears Small 6”	1	1	1
Eye Pad Dressing with Bandage Sterile	2	3	4
Foil Blanket Adult Size	1	2	3
First Aid Guidance Leaflet	1	1	1

2.5 Managing an Incident

Providing safe, prompt and effective first aid to a casualty can only be done through careful management of an incident.

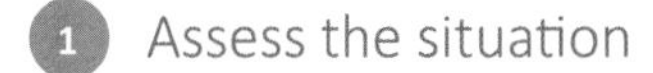

1. Assess the situation
2. Make the area as safe as possible
3. Find out what has happened
4. Take control
5. Send for help
6. Begin providing first aid

‘Providing safe, prompt and effective first aid to a casualty can only be done through careful management of an incident’

Unresponsive Casualty

3.1 Assessing a Casualty

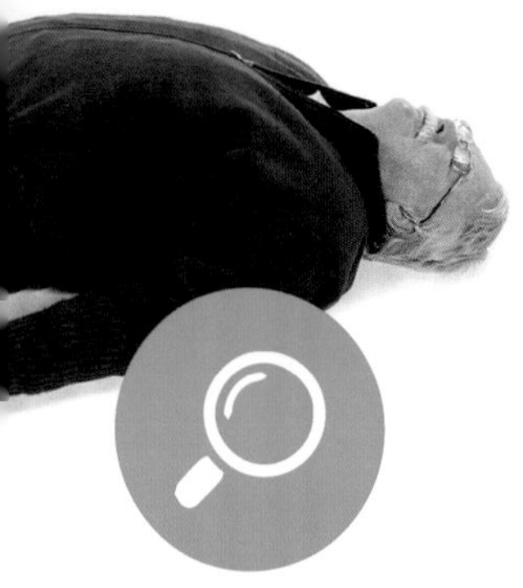

Once you have established that it is safe to approach your casualty, you now need to establish what's wrong with the casualty. This is done through a series of logical surveys based upon the priorities of first aid.

Your priorities as a first aider are to open the airway of the casualty and check their breathing. Once that is established and maintained we can then turn our attention to see if the casualty is bleeding or has any burns. Once these are managed we can finally investigate and treat any breaks that may have occurred.

3.2 The Primary Survey

DRAB

By starting our assessment and treatment of an unresponsive casualty with the primary survey we are ensuring that we find and deal with the most life threatening conditions first and are not distracted by any non life threatening conditions.

Remembering and using the acronym DRAB will ensure you perform the actions of the primary survey in the correct sequence.

'Using the acronym DRAB will ensure you perform the actions of the primary survey in the correct sequence'

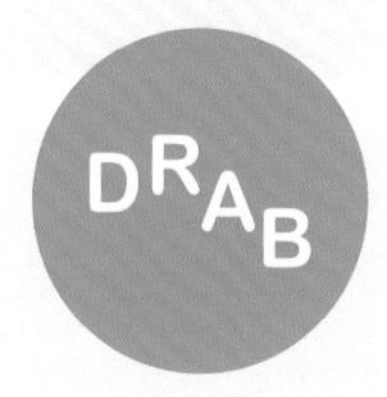

D

Danger

Check the area is safe, if necessary and if it is safe to do so remove any hazards.

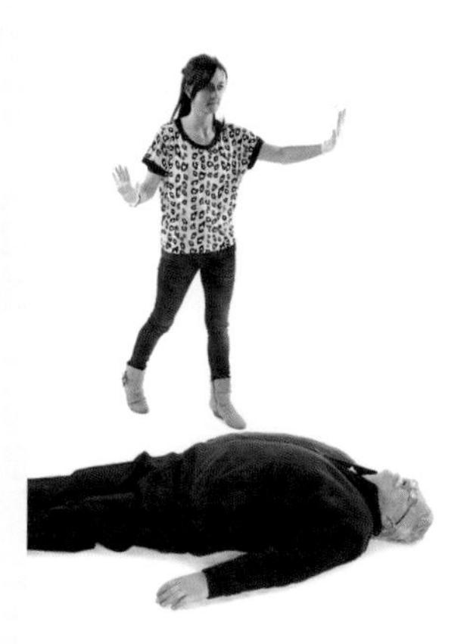

R

Response

Check to ensure the casualty is responsive. Gently squeeze the shoulders and ask them loudly 'Are you alright?'

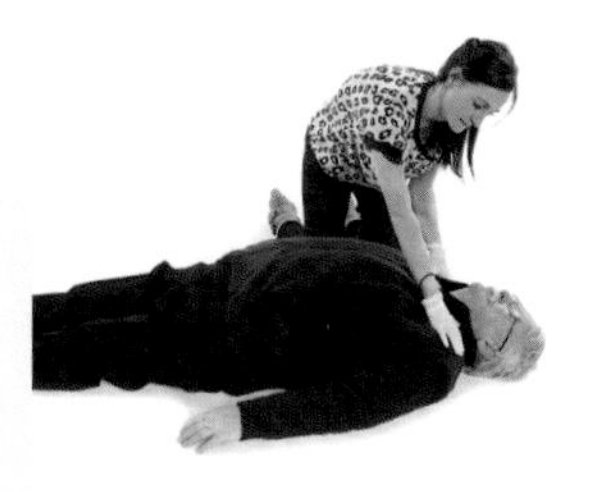

A

Airway

If there is no response, open the airway using the head tilt/chin lift method.

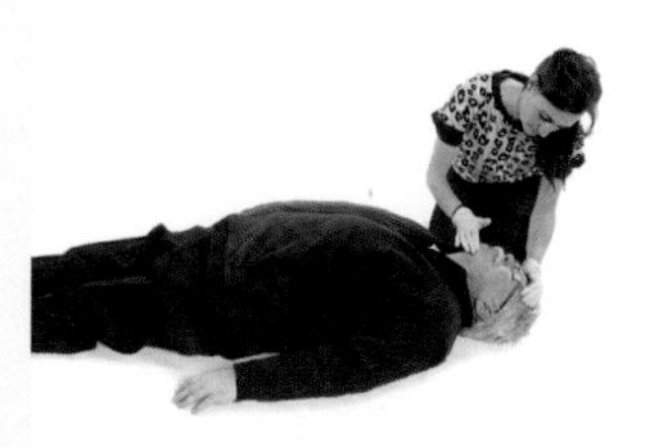

B

Breathing

Check, look and listen for up to 10 seconds for normal breathing.

1 breathe in 10 seconds is not normal.
2-3/10 secs is normal.

If breathing normally:
Place them in the recovery position (page 13).

If NOT breathing normally:
Arrange for an ambulance, ask for an AED and begin CPR.

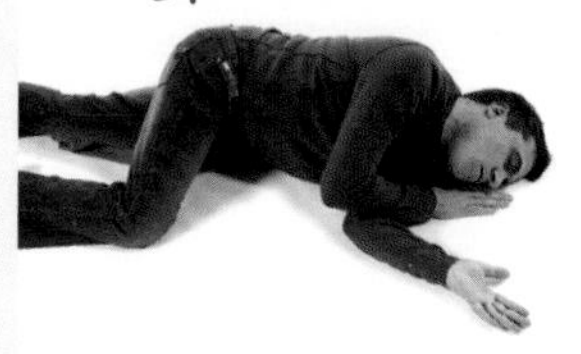

Unresponsive Casualty

3.3 Secondary Survey

Once you have performed a successful primary survey and are happy that the casualty is breathing normally and not suffering from any major blood loss, you can begin to perform a secondary survey. During this methodical survey you are looking for other non life threatening injuries or illnesses. This is often referred to as the 'head to toe' or 'top to toe' survey.

Use all your senses to look, listen and feel your way down the casualty's body, without any unnecessary movement of the casualty. All the time, ask yourself, bystanders and the patient some simple questions.

- **What happened?** This will establish the history of the event leading up to the illness or injury.
- **What can I see?** This will give you vital signs of any injuries (bruising, swelling deformity, etc.).
- **Listen** to what the casualty is telling you. These are the symptoms of the injury or illness the casualty is suffering from (location and type of pain, nausea, feeling hot or cold, etc.).

Head to Toe Survey

1 Head and Neck

- Continue to monitor the casualty's breathing and circulation.
- Run your hands across the head and around the back of the neck checking for fluid, lumps, bumps, irregularity or deformity. Check your hands.
- Look in the ears for fluid (see head injuries) and talk to the casualty, looking for a response.
- Look in both eyes, compare and contrast pupil size, look for discolouration or foreign objects.
- Assess the skin. Is it normal in colour? Pale or flushed? Cold or hot? Wet or dry? The skin will tell you if there is something wrong.

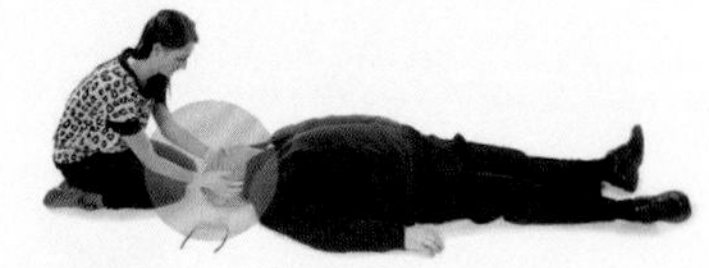

2 Chest

- Run your hands across the shoulders and collar bones, compare and contrast. Loosen any clothing around the neck area to aid breathing and circulation.

- Can the casualty breathe easily? Feel both sides of the chest, looking for equal pain free movement from the casualty.

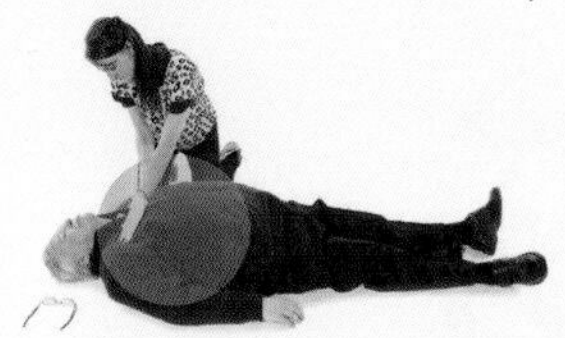

3 Stomach and Hips

- Gently feel the stomach area looking for pain or discomfort.
- Do the same with the hips (but **DO NOT** rock them) whilst looking for signs of bleeding or incontinence.

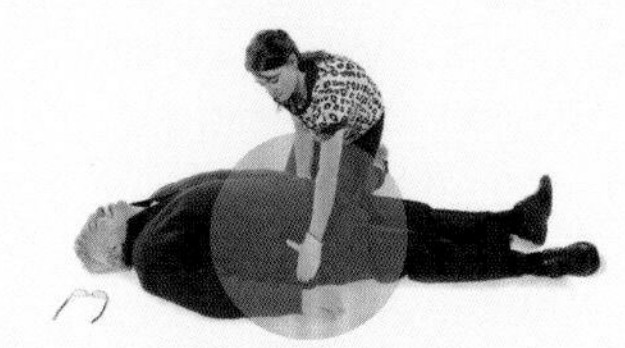

4 Arms

- Run your hands along each arm feeling and looking for lumps, bumps, irregularity and deformity.
- If the casualty can move their arms, hands and fingers, ask them to do so. Check the fingertips for signs of cyanosis.

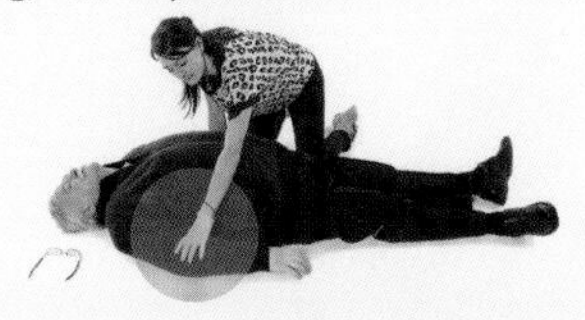

5 Legs

- Run your hands along each leg feeling and looking for lumps, bumps, irregularity and deformity.
- If the casualty can move their legs, hands and fingers, ask them to do so.
- If possible check the toes for signs of cyanosis.

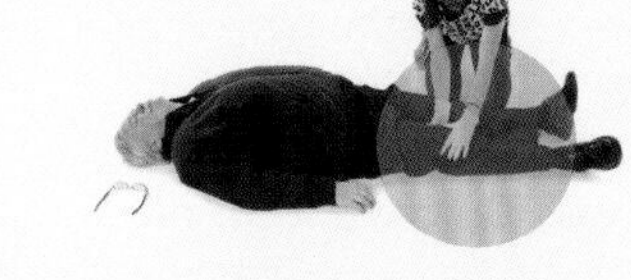

6 Medical Clues

Your casualty may have some additional clues hidden around their body which may help you ascertain what is wrong with them.

- Pockets. Be aware of needles! Check inside for ID or medication (inhalers, EpiPens or GTN sprays).
- Medic Alert Bracelets. Check for bracelets inscribed with any medical conditions the casualty may suffer from (such as anaphylaxis, epilepsy, or diabetes).

'If safe to do so, leave the casualty in the position that you found them and begin your survey at the head and slowly work your way down the body to the toes'

3.4 The Recovery Position

If we discover a casualty who is unresponsive and breathing normally, we place them in the recovery position. We do this to manage their airway, prevent the tongue from falling towards the back of the throat and protecting their airway from vomit.

1 Perform your primary survey (DRAB). Kneel down next to the casualty, roughly level with the chest. Grab hold of the arm that is closest to you, bend the elbow and allow the hand to rest palm upwards.

2 Grab the arm furthest from you, bring it towards you, hold the hand with your hand, palm to palm and place the back of the casualty's hand on the casualty's cheek.

3 With your free hand, reach across to the casualty's leg that is furthest from you and pull it up from behind the knee, bending the leg so that the foot is flat on the floor. Keep hold of the hand on the casualty's cheek and then place your other hand on top of their knee.

4 Push down on the knee towards you and the casualty will begin to roll onto his side. Allow the casualty to roll all the way over. Adjust the upper leg at the hip so that the knee is bent at right angles. Tilt the head back to extend the airway.

5 Now call 999/112 and ask for an ambulance if this hasn't been done yet. Continue to monitor breathing and circulation regularly. Keep the casualty warm and be prepared to resuscitate if they stop breathing.

Pregnant woman - put them on their Left hand side to avoid pressing on their vera cava inferior which runs down their RHS.

3.5 CPR Adult

Chain of Survival

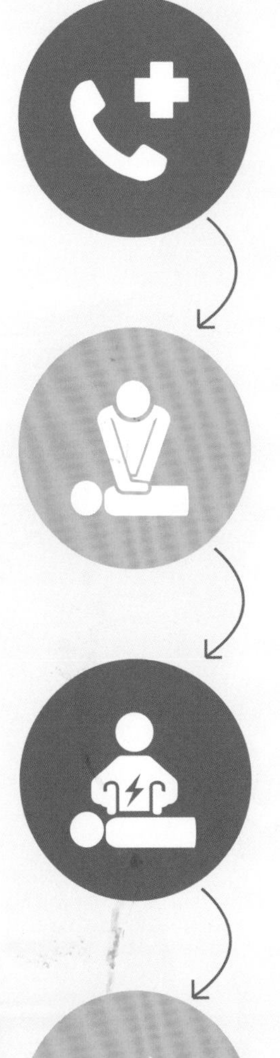

Call for Help

It is vital that the ambulance service has been called as soon as possible. For every minute that goes by the chance of survival of a victim of cardiac arrest reduces by about 10%. Call 999/112 yourself or even better ask a bystander to do it for you whilst you begin CPR.

Early CPR

Effective CPR, with an emphasis on chest compressions, should commence as soon as possible after the collapse of the victim. CPR will ensure oxygenated blood reaches the vital organs including the heart and brain. CPR will also help keep the heart in a shockable rhythm like ventricular fibrillation for when the defibrillator arrives.

Early Defibrillation

The sooner the victim of cardiac arrest can receive a life saving shock of electricity from a defibrillator the greater their chance of survival becomes.

This link in the chain is the most important determinant of survival and supports the call for greater availability of public access defibrillators.

Early ALS/Post Resuscitation Care

The final link is the care administered by medical professionals, such as paramedics, doctors and nurses who will provide advanced life support techniques to increase the victims chance of survival beyond hospital.

Unresponsive Casualty
CPR Adult

CPR Step by Step

If we discover a casualty who is unresponsive and NOT breathing normally, we have to perform CPR, cardiopulmonary resuscitation. The purpose of CPR is to maintain oxygenated blood to the vital organs and to maintain the heart in a shockable rhythm before the arrival of a defibrillator.

Perform your primary survey (DRAB). Kneel down next to the casualty, roughly level with the chest.

If you are alone, leave the casualty to phone for an ambulance and grab a defibrillator. If you have a bystander present send them to do it for you.

If the casualty is not breathing normally begin CPR. Give 30 chest compressions and 2 rescue breaths.

Continue giving cycles of 30 chest compressions and 2 rescue breaths until:
Help arrives, the casualty begins to regain responsiveness and starts breathing normally again or you become too exhausted to continue performing CPR.

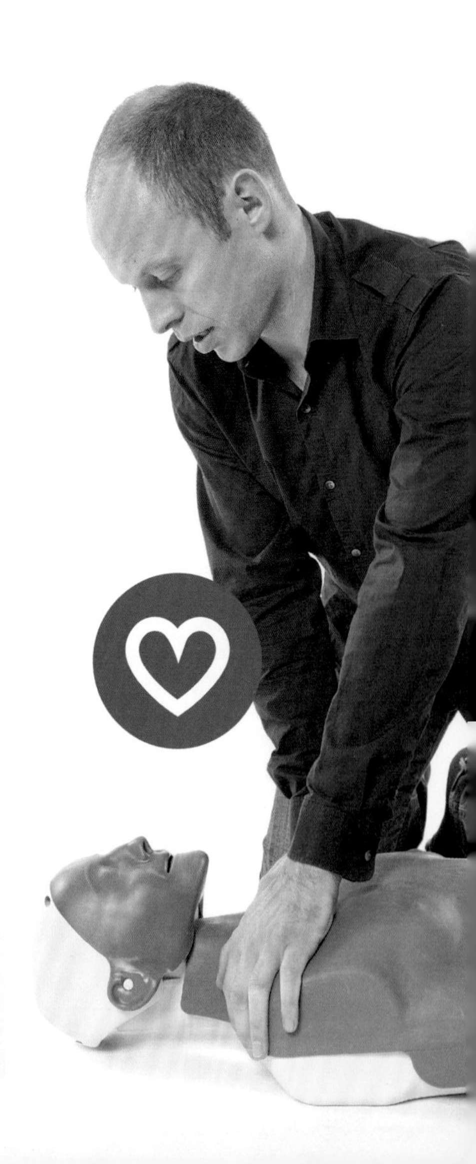

Chest Compressions

- Place the heel of one hand in the centre of the casualty's chest.
- Place the other hand on top of your first and interlock your fingers.
- Lock your elbows and begin to compress the chest 30 times at a rate of 100-120 compressions a minute at a depth of 5-6 cms.

Rescue Breaths

- Place the palm of one hand on the casualty's forehead.
- Place the other hand under the casualty's chin and tilt the head back, extending the airway.
- Keep your hand under the chin and use your other hand to pinch the casualty's nose.
- Open your mouth, make a seal around the casualty's mouth with yours and blow (use a barrier if available), watching the rise and fall of the casualty's chest.
- Blow no more than a second and repeat.

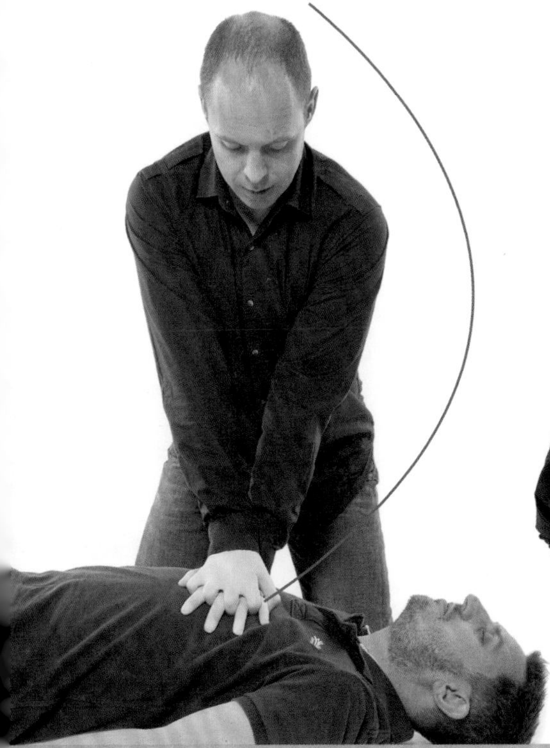

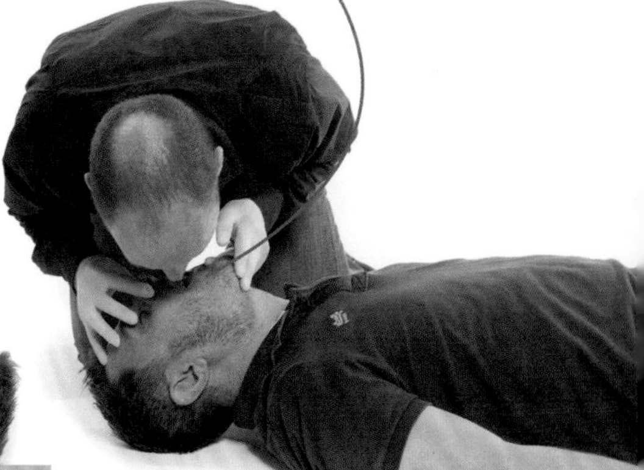

'Give 30 chest compressions and 2 rescue breaths'

Unresponsive Casualty

3.6 CPR Child (1 year to puberty)

If we discover a child who is unresponsive and NOT breathing normally, we have to perform CPR, cardiopulmonary resuscitation. The steps you are to follow are very similar to adult CPR with a couple of modifications to make them more appropriate to children. However the same steps for adults can be followed for resuscitation for children; it is far better to use the adult BLS sequence for resuscitation of a child than to do nothing. A child is aged between one and puberty.

Chest Compressions and Rescue Breaths

Rescue Breaths

- Place the palm of one hand on the child's forehead. Place the other hand under the child's chin and tilt the head back, extending the airway. Keep your hand under the chin and use your other hand to pinch the casualty's nose.
- Open your mouth; make a seal around the child's mouth with yours and blow, watching the rise and fall of the child's chest. Blow no more than one second and repeat.

Chest Compressions

- Place one or two hands in the centre of the child's chest.
- Compress the chest by at least one-third of its depth at a rate of 100-120 compressions per minute.

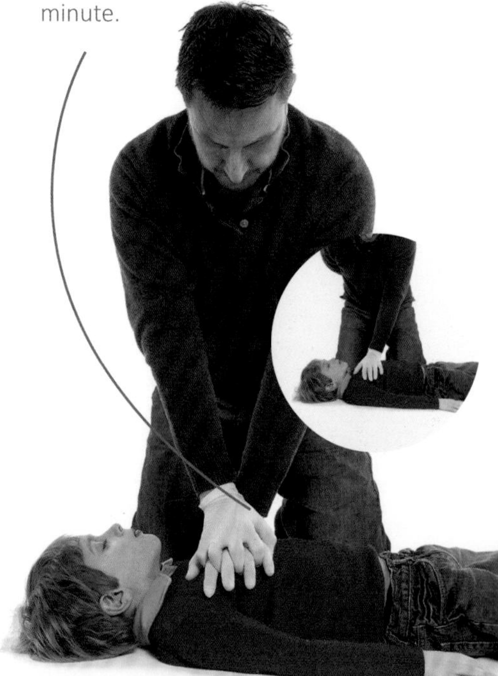

'A child is aged between one and puberty'

CPR Step by Step

1

Perform the primary survey (DRAB); tap the child's shoulder. Kneel down next to the child, roughly level with the chest. If CPR is to be performed on the child, the decision must be made within 10 seconds of starting the initial assessment. If there is any doubt after this time, start CPR.

2

If you are alone, and the child is NOT breathing normally, activate the speaker function on your mobile and dial 999/112 for an ambulance whilst providing care to the casualty. If no mobile phone is available, give 5 initial rescue breaths followed by 1 minute of CPR then dial 999/112 for an ambulance. Grab an AED with paediatric electrode pads (AEDs cannot be used on infants). If you have a bystander present send them to do it immediately.

Upon your return/once the ambulance has been arranged, continue giving 30 chest compressions followed by 2 rescue breaths.

Continue giving cycles of 30 chest compressions and 2 rescue breaths until: Help arrives, the casualty begins to regain responsiveness and starts breathing normally again, you become too exhausted to continue performing CPR.

3.7 CPR Infant (under 1 year)

If we discover an infant who is unresponsive and NOT breathing normally, we still have to perform CPR, cardiopulmonary resuscitation. Many people are concerned about performing CPR on such a small person for fear of 'hurting' them however this is the infant's best chance of survival. The steps you are to follow are very similar to adult CPR with a couple of modifications. An infant is less than one year old.

Chest Compressions and Rescue Breaths

Chest Compressions

- Place two fingers in the centre of the infant's chest and compress the chest by at least one-third of its depth at a rate of 100-120 compressions per minute.

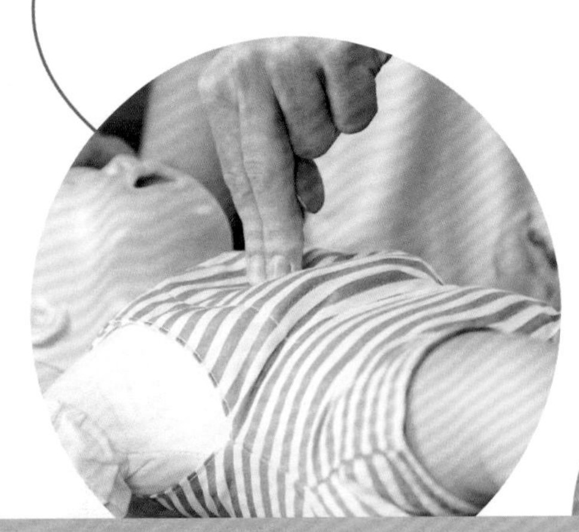

Rescue Breaths

- Place the palm of one hand on the infant's head in a neutral position, extending the airway but be careful not to overextend.
- Open your mouth; make a seal around the infant's mouth and nose and blow gently, watching the rise and fall of the infant's chest. **DO NOT** overinflate the infant's lungs. Blow no more than a second and repeat.

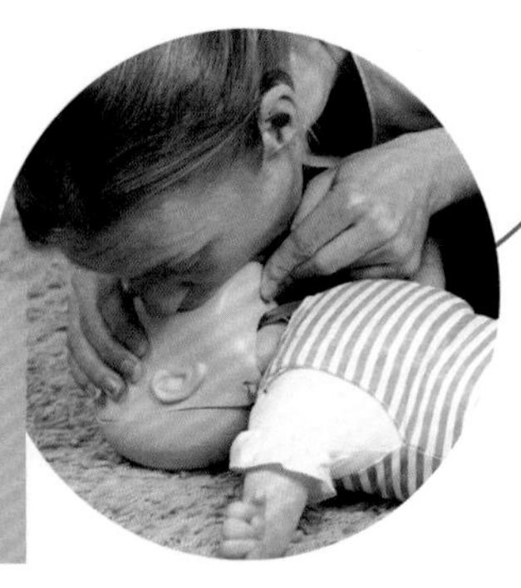

'DO NOT overinflate the infant's lungs'

1

Perform your primary survey (DRAB); tap the infant's foot. Kneel down next to the infant, roughly level with the chest.

If you are alone, and the infant is NOT breathing normally, activate the speaker function on your mobile and dial 999/112 for an ambulance whilst providing care to the casualty. If no mobile phone is available, give 5 initial rescue breaths followed by 1 minute of CPR then dial 999/112 for an ambulance. If you have a bystander present send them immediately to call 999/112 for an ambulance.

Upon your return/once the ambulance has been arranged, continue 30 chest compressions followed by 2 rescue breaths until help arrives, the infant begins to regain responsiveness and starts breathing normally again or you become too exhausted to continue performing CPR.

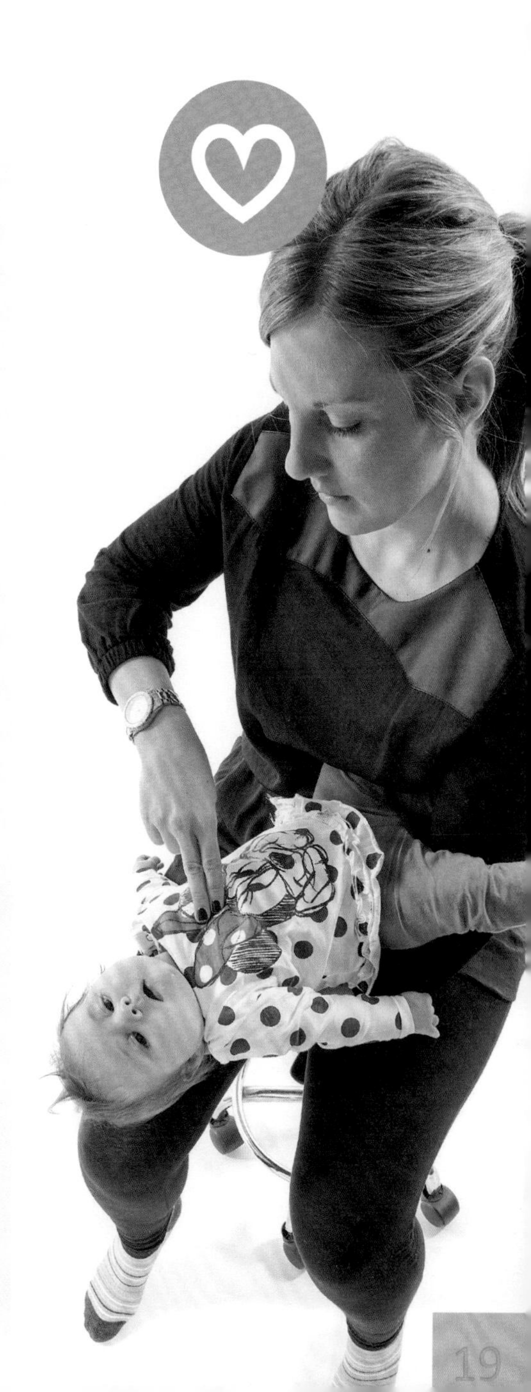

3.8 Use of an AED - Step by Step

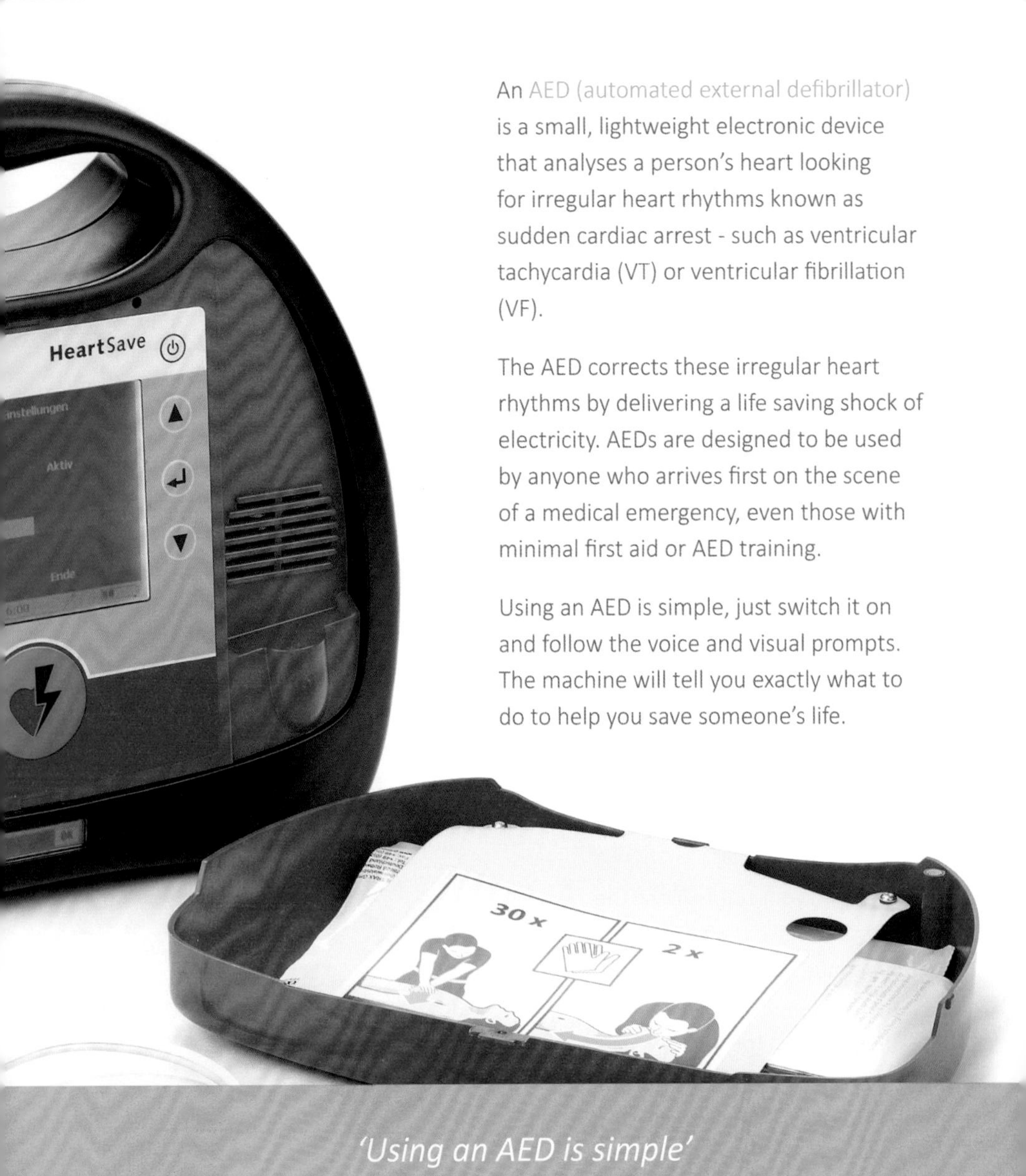

An AED (automated external defibrillator) is a small, lightweight electronic device that analyses a person's heart looking for irregular heart rhythms known as sudden cardiac arrest - such as ventricular tachycardia (VT) or ventricular fibrillation (VF).

The AED corrects these irregular heart rhythms by delivering a life saving shock of electricity. AEDs are designed to be used by anyone who arrives first on the scene of a medical emergency, even those with minimal first aid or AED training.

Using an AED is simple, just switch it on and follow the voice and visual prompts. The machine will tell you exactly what to do to help you save someone's life.

'Using an AED is simple'

Do not defibrillate a baby < 1 year.

Step by Step

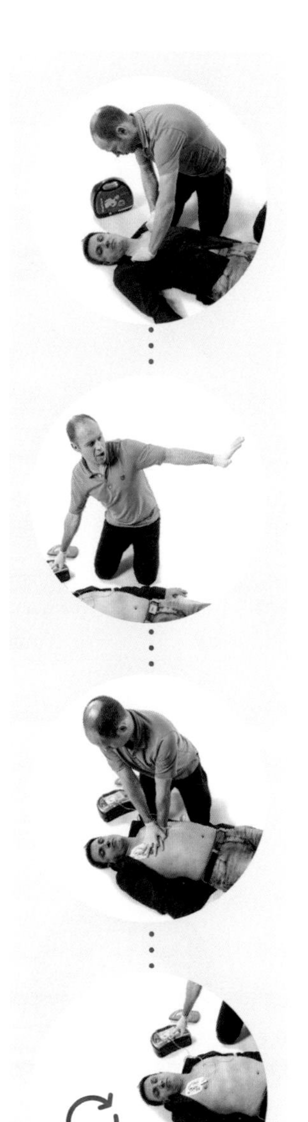

Switch on the AED and follow the voice and visual prompts.

Remove the casualty's clothing from their upper chest.

Take out the electrode pads from the packaging and place on the patient's bare chest as directed by the AED.

Once both electrode pads are in place the AED will begin to analyse the casualty's heart rhythm. Ensure no one is touching the casualty during analysis.

Shock advised:

Make sure everyone is clear of the casualty and push the flashing shock button to deliver the life saving shock of electricity. Follow the prompts from the AED and continue delivering CPR.

No shock advised:

Follow the prompts from the AED and continue delivering CPR.

Continue with CPR for two minutes.

After two minutes the AED will re-analyse the casualty's heart rhythm to see if a shock needs to be delivered or not. This sequence of two minutes of CPR then analysis will continue until professional help arrives.

with children, if pads too big to put in standard places, can do front + back.

Breathing Problems

4.1 Airway Obstruction

It is vital to our survival that we keep our airways open (nose, mouth, throat and lungs). As air travels through the airway to our lungs, oxygen gets transferred into our blood. Blockages to the airway are life threatening emergencies and must be dealt with immediately.

A blockage can be internal, such as swallowing an object or swelling as a result of a burn or allergic reaction or it can be external as a result of strangulation or hanging.

'If the casualty becomes unresponsive begin CPR immediately'

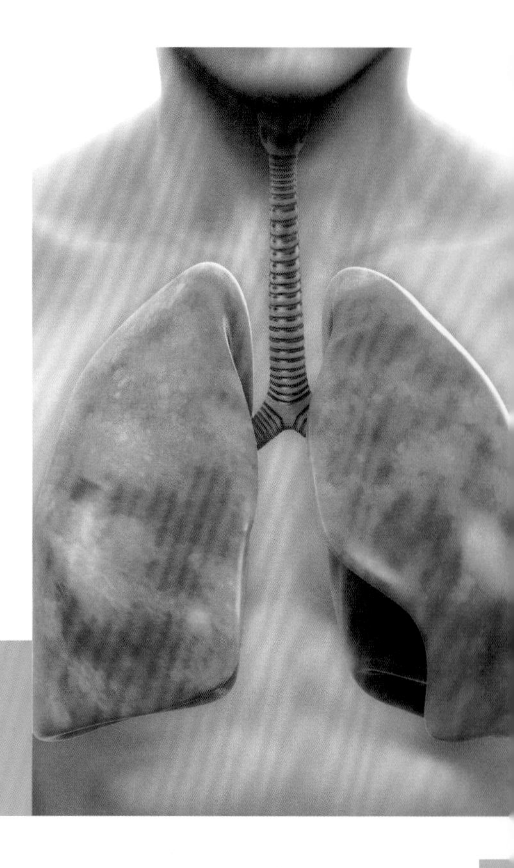

4.2 Choking Adult

Objects can become partially or fully stuck in the throat. This causes the muscles in the throat to spasm and breathing difficult or impossible.

Partial blockage

If a casualty has a 'partial blockage' they are able to speak, cough and breathe. Your job as a first aider is to encourage them to keep calm and cough. The idea being that the obstruction frees itself.

Full blockage

If however the casualty cannot speak, cough or breathe then a 'full blockage' has occurred and this blockage needs clearing before the casualty loses responsiveness.

Treatment

Encourage the casualty to bend forward from the waist and support them with one hand.

Back Blows

With the other hand give up to 5 back blows with the heel of your hand, between the casualty's shoulder blades.

If the obstruction isn't cleared, stand behind the casualty, place both your arms around them and encourage them to lean forward.

Abdominal Thrusts

With one fist placed between the belly button and the bottom of the breastbone and the other fist on top of the first, pull sharply inwards and upwards. Repeat this sharp motion up to 5 times. Medical attention should be advised if this technique is used due to the possibility of internal damage.

Check the casualty's mouth for obstructions and repeat 5 back blows then 5 abdominal thrusts, up to three times. If the obstruction still has not cleared call for an ambulance 999/112 and continue until help arrives or the casualty becomes unresponsive. If unresponsive, begin CPR immediately.

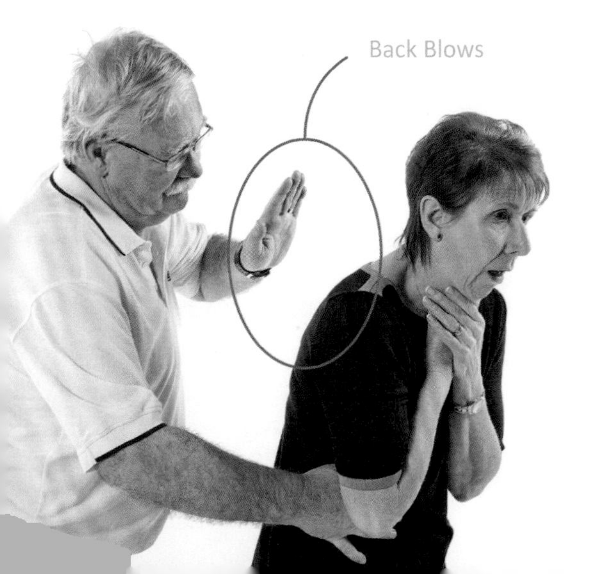

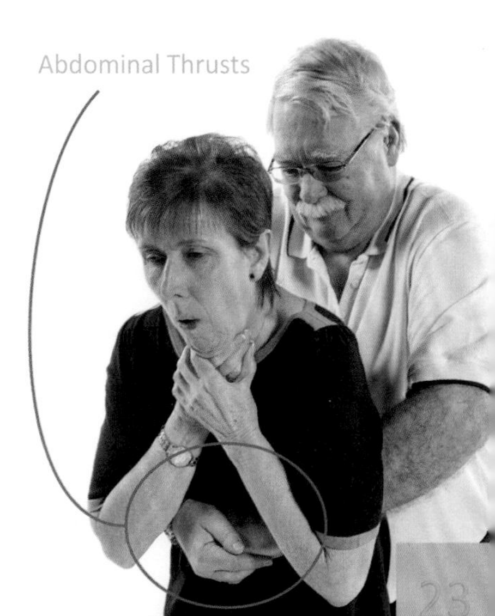

4.3 Choking Child & Infant

Children and infants can easily choke on small objects and food. In these instances you will need to act immediately to prevent the child from panicking and/or going unresponsive.

Partial Blockage

If a child or an infant has a 'partial blockage' they are able to speak, cough and breathe. Your job as a first aider is to encourage them to keep calm and cough. The idea being that the obstruction frees itself.

Full Blockage

If however the child or infant cannot speak, cough or breathe then a 'full blockage' has occurred.

'If the child becomes unresponsive, begin CPR immediately'

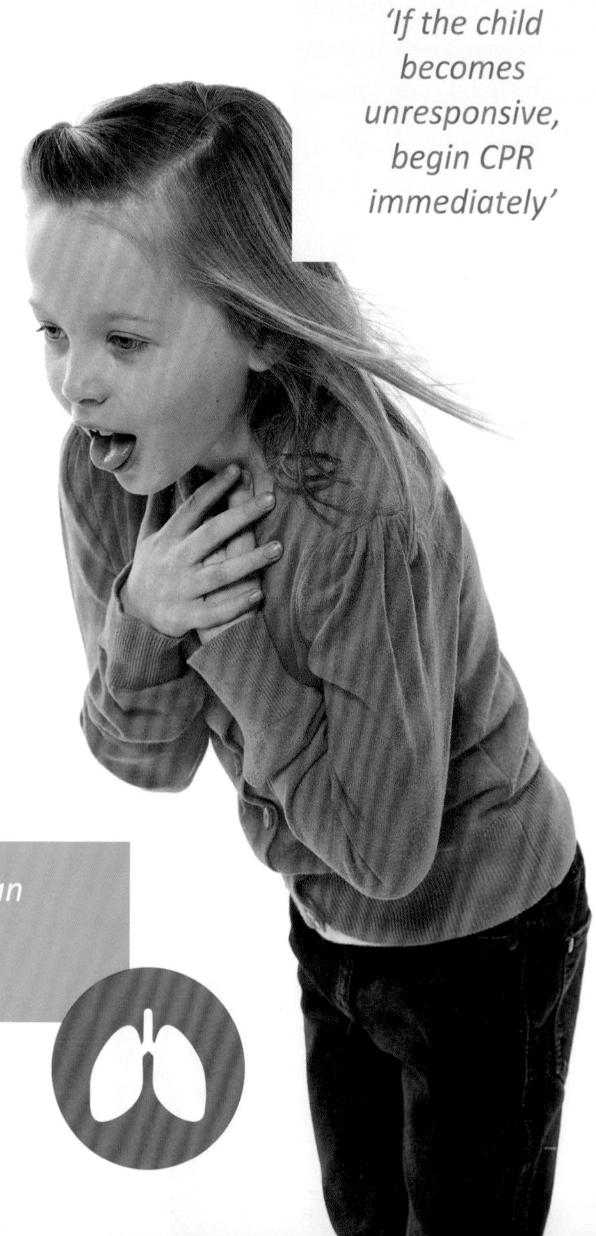

'Children and infants can easily choke on small objects and food'

Treatment Child (1 year to puberty)

Encourage the child to bend forward from the waist or bend them over your knee so that their head is lower than their chest.

Back Blows
With the other hand give up to 5 back blows with the heel of your hand, between the child's shoulder blades.

If the obstruction hasn't cleared, stand or kneel behind the child, place both your arms around their waist and encourage them to lean forward.

Abdominal Thrusts
With one fist placed between the belly button and the bottom of the breastbone and the other fist on top of the first, pull sharply inwards and upwards. Repeat this sharp motion up to 5 times. Medical attention should be advised if this technique is used due to the possibility of internal damage.

Check the child's mouth for obstructions and repeat 5 back blows then 5 abdominal thrusts, up to three times. If the obstruction still has not cleared call for an ambulance 999/112 and continue until help arrives or the child becomes unresponsive. If unresponsive, begin CPR immediately.

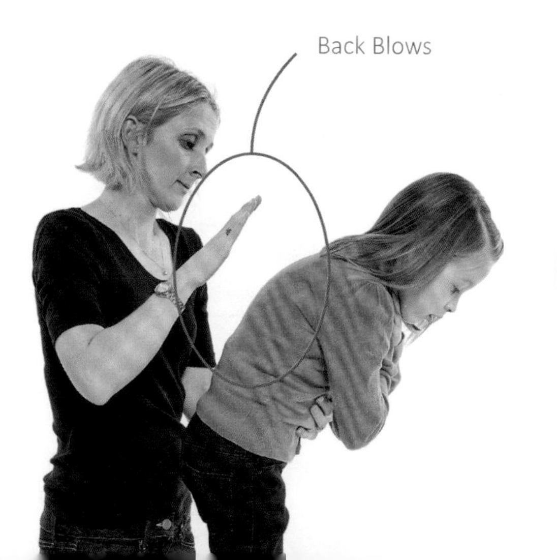

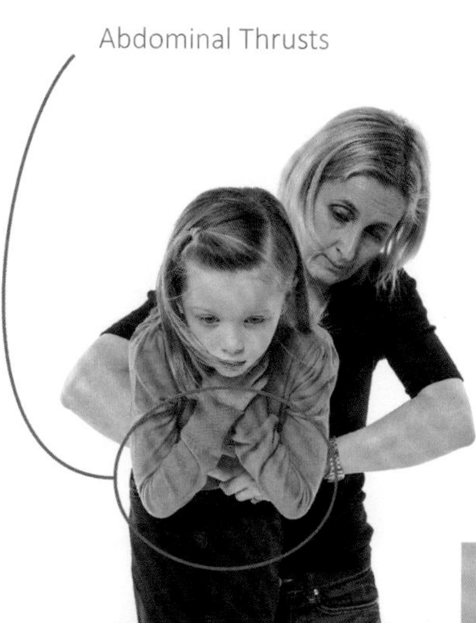

Breathing Problems
Choking Child & Infant

Treatment Infant (under 1 year)

Lay the infant face down along your forearm so that their head is lower than their chest.

Back Blow

With one hand give up to 5 back blows with the heel of your hand, between the infant's shoulder blades. Check the infant's mouth for obstructions between each back blow.

Chest Thrusts

If the obstruction hasn't cleared, turn the infant over onto their back. Place two fingers on the breastbone and thrust sharply inwards and upwards, towards the infant's head. Medical attention should be advised if this technique is used due to the possibility of internal damage. Repeat up to 5 times, checking for obstructions after each thrust.

Check the infant's mouth for obstructions and repeat 5 back blows then 5 chest thrusts, up to three times.

If the obstruction still has not cleared call for an ambulance 999/112 and continue until help arrives or the infant becomes unresponsive. If unresponsive, begin CPR immediately.

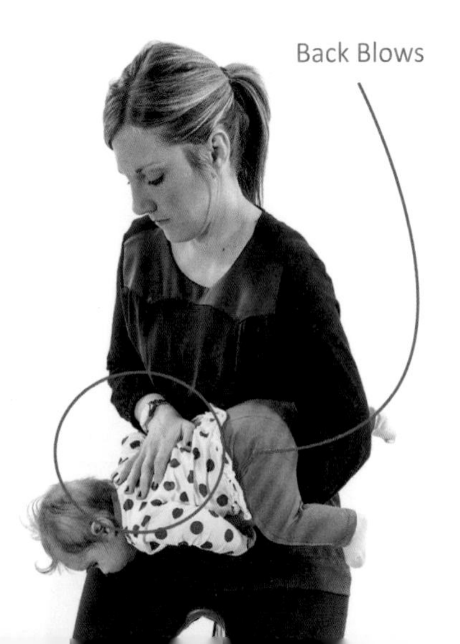

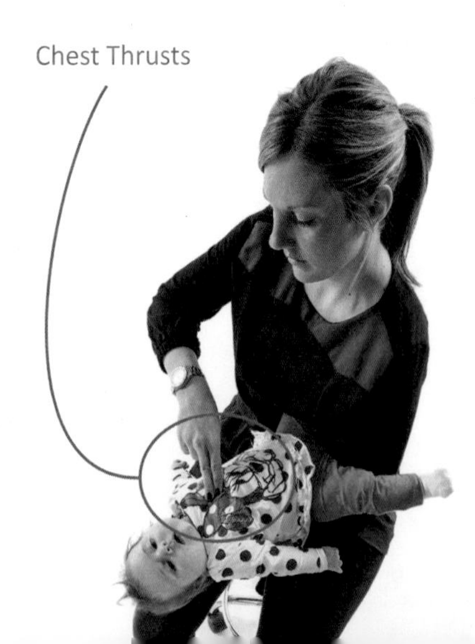

4.4 Drowning

Around 400 people drown in the UK each year. Drowning occurs when water enters the lungs causing the throat to go into spasm blocking the airway. The actual amount of water that enters the lungs maybe small but the irritation it causes in the lungs leads to a build up of fluid which prevents the efficient transfer of oxygen from the lungs into the blood. This may be immediate or it may take up to 72 hours to occur, this is known as secondary drowning.

Treatment

If you suspect someone has drowned and it is safe to do so rescue them from the water.

If they are responsive:
Lie them down with their head lower-most and tilted to one side to allow water to drain out of their mouth, keep them warm to prevent Hypothermia, and call 999/112 because of the risk of secondary drowning.

If they are unresponsive:
Breathing normally:
Place in the recovery position and keep warm, call 999/112 and monitor.
Not breathing normally:
Begin CPR but with 5 initial breaths before you start compressions. After performing CPR for one minute, if you are alone, call 999/112 for an ambulance and then return and continue CPR as normal until an AED arrives.

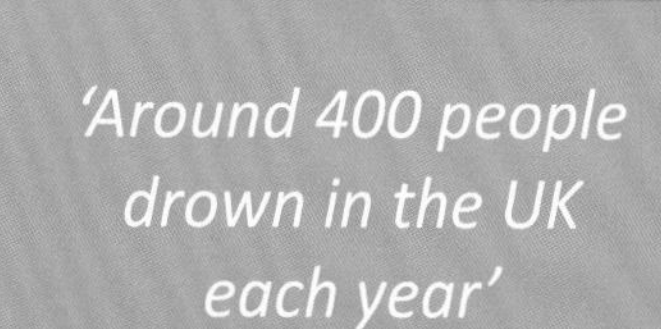

'Around 400 people drown in the UK each year'

Breathing Problems

4.5 Inhalation of Fumes

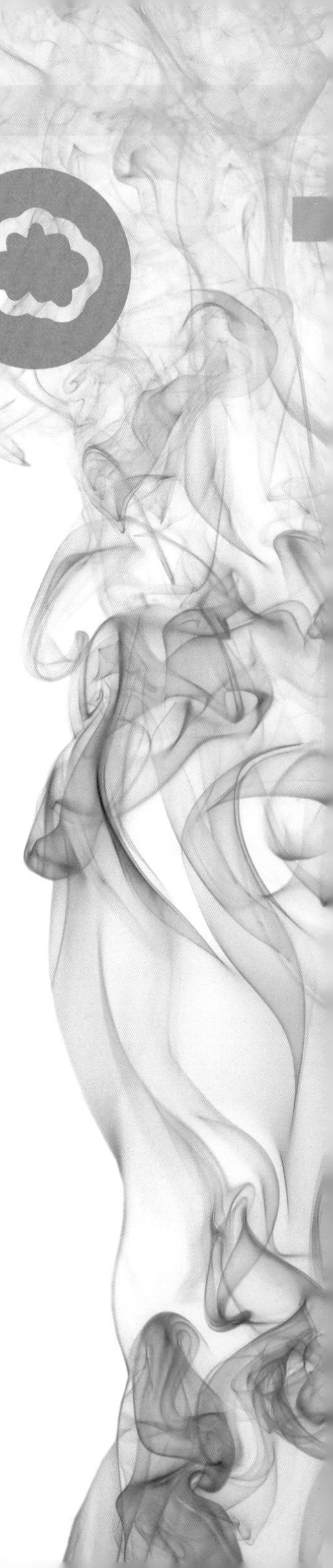

Like water, smoke, gases, toxic fumes or vapours can enter the lungs and prevent oxygen from reaching the blood. Some of these fumes are visible to the naked eye or can be smelt, others cannot such as carbon monoxide, so it is imperative that you consider your own safety if you believe that a casualty has suffered from inhalation of fumes.

Recognition

Carbon Monoxide
Difficulty breathing, headache, nausea.

Solvents
Impaired level of responsiveness, headache, vomiting, smell of solvent on breath, could lead to cardiac arrest.

Smoke
Coughing, burning sensation in the throat, soot around mouth and nose.

Treatment

Move casualty into an area with fresh air, if it is safe to do so.

Encourage casualty to breathe normally.

Treat any burns as appropriate and be prepared to resuscitate.

Call 999/112 for medical assistance.

Wounds & Bleeding

5.1 Types of Wounds

A wound is an injury to the skin. Wounds carry different classifications depending on what causes the injury. Be aware that wounds carry the risk of infection.

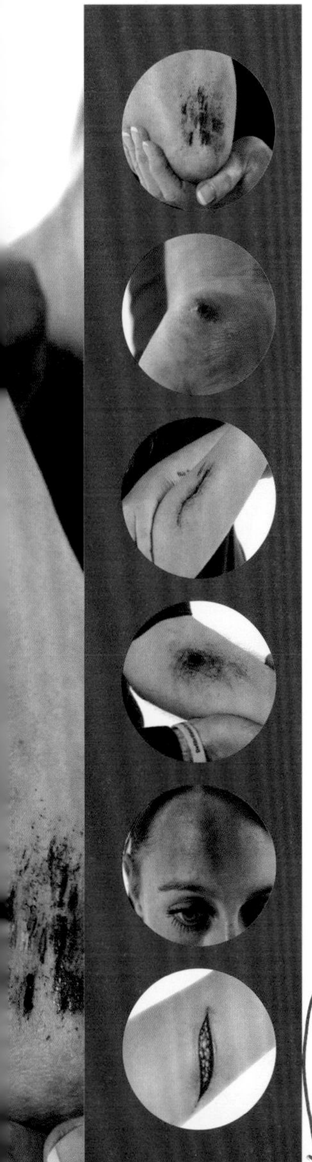

Abrasion

Typically known as a graze, this wound is superficial and involves the removal of the top layers of skin. As grazes are often caused by friction there is a high risk of foreign objects being introduced to the wound which could lead to infection.

Puncture

Anything that enters into the skin is classed as a puncture wound. The wound itself may appear quite small but the depth can lead to extensive internal damage and an increased risk of infection.

Incision

A 'clean' cut from a sharp edge like a knife. Incisions can be deep and cause increased blood loss and damage to underlying soft tissues.

Velocity

A small entry wound and very large exit wound typify this wound caused by a high velocity projectile like a bullet. As the projectile passes through the body it brings with it a high risk of infection as well as the ability to damage internal organs potentially leading to massive blood loss.

Contusion

Better known as a bruise, a contused wound is a break in the capillaries of the skin caused by a blunt instrument like a hammer. This can lead to unseen damage to bones or tissues.

Laceration

A laceration of the skin is a rough tear which may carry a risk of infection as well as being difficult to treat as the wound is not as neat as an incision.

seek further medical attention if bruise on arms, legs > palm of hand size ; on body > 50p piece size

5.2 Controlling Bleeding

The amount of blood loss from a wound will depend on which blood vessels have been damaged.

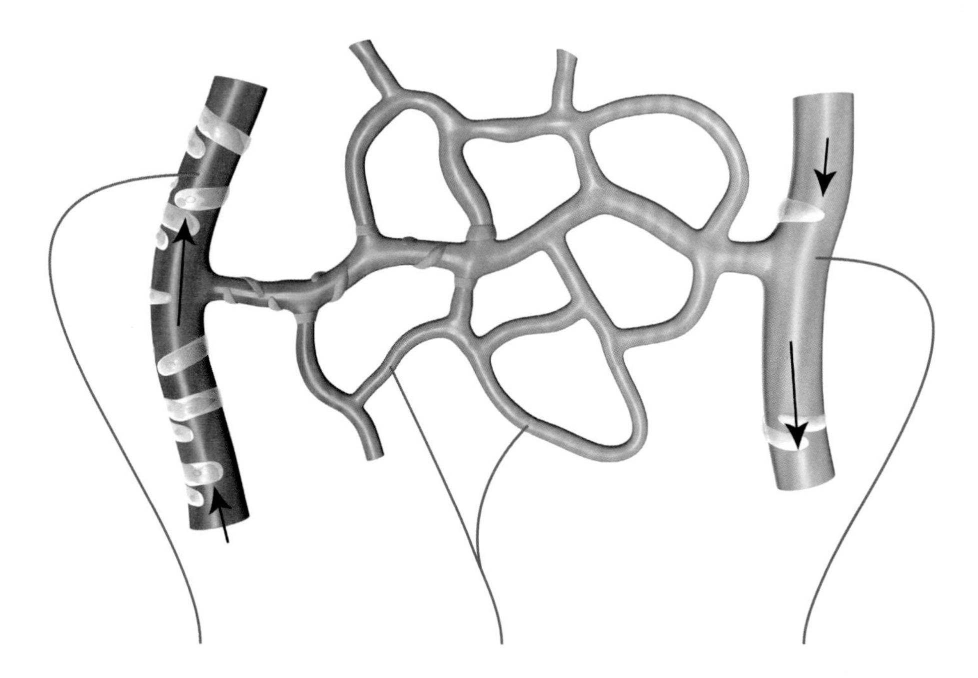

Arteries

Produce bright red highly oxygenated blood which 'spurts' out in time with each heartbeat. A lot of blood loss occurs when arteries have been damaged.

Capillaries

All wounds have some blood loss from the capillaries. This type of bleeding 'oozes' at the site of the wound and usually only a small amount of blood loss results.

Veins

This blood loss 'gushes' rather than spurts as the blood is under less pressure as it returns to the heart. The blood is darker red in colour but the loss can still be significant.

Treatment

As a first aider it is a priority to reduce blood loss, minimise infection, prevent and treat for shock. This can be done in three simple steps:

Focus on applying direct pressure to the wound. Ask the casualty to do it themselves until you can apply a clean, non fluffy sterile dressing. If there is an embedded object apply pressure either side of the object.

Depending on the location of the wound, sit or lay the casualty down. If the bleeding is severe, treat for the prevention of shock by laying the casualty down and elevating the legs. Keep the casualty warm.

If bleeding continues through the first dressing, apply another one. If bleeding continues remove both and start again. Ensuring pressure is being applied directly over the wound. If bleeding cannot be controlled by applying pressure to the wound you may need to consider a tourniquet or haemostatic dressing (only attempt this if you are suitably trained and the correct equipment is available).

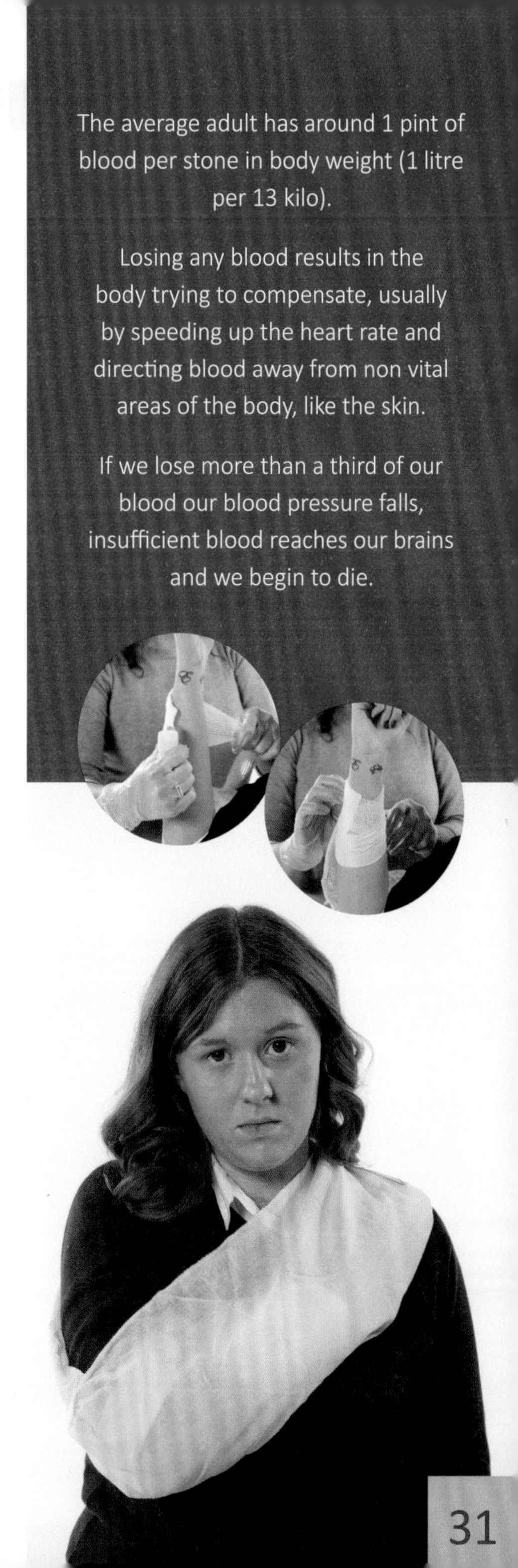

The average adult has around 1 pint of blood per stone in body weight (1 litre per 13 kilo).

Losing any blood results in the body trying to compensate, usually by speeding up the heart rate and directing blood away from non vital areas of the body, like the skin.

If we lose more than a third of our blood our blood pressure falls, insufficient blood reaches our brains and we begin to die.

Wounds & Bleeding

5.3 Catastrophic Bleeding

Recognition

When we have a casualty with a catastrophic bleed, we adjust the primary survey to DRCAB (C - Manage any catastrophic bleeding: Apply tourniquet and/or haemostatic dressing). A bleed would be classed as a catastrophic bleed if it meets any of the following criteria;

- There is a traumatic amputation of the arm or leg.
- There is pulsating or severe bleeding from a wound.
- Blood is pooling quickly or in large quantities on the ground.
- Bandages or makeshift bandages used to cover the wound are ineffective or becoming soaked with blood.

D
Danger
R
Response
C
Catastrophic Bleeding
A
Airway
B
Breathing

Haemostatic dressings

Haemostatic dressings save lives by quickly clotting the blood of a casualty which reduces blood loss. Although they are simple to use, additional training is recommended by the HSE for first aiders who may need to apply a haemostatic dressing. Haemostatic dressings are typically used for severe wounds to the torso, neck or groin areas.

Haemostatic dressings

How to use

Simple steps to apply a haemostatic dressing are:

- Pinpoint the exact source of the bleeding.
- Apply direct pressure to the bleeding and use a normal sterile bandage to absorb any excess blood from the wound if necessary.
- Tightly pack the entire wound with the haemostatic dressing.
- Apply direct pressure to the packed dressing for a minimum of 5 minutes. Repeat this step if bleeding continues.
- Once the bleeding is under control, leave the haemostatic dressing in place and cover with a normal sterile dressing.
- Ensure the packaging from the dressing is given to the medical professionals upon arrival.

Tourniquets

Tourniquets are used to minimise blood flow by being applied and tightened around a severely wounded limb. By incorrectly applying a tourniquet, the veins can be squashed instead of the arteries, therefore increasing blood loss and worsening the situation. Additional training is recommended by the HSE for first aiders who may need to apply a tourniquet. A tourniquet should only be used in a life threatening situation where the bleeding cannot be controlled by direct pressure.

How to use

There are several tourniquet types available on the market and each should be used in line with the manufacturer's application guidelines. The general steps to apply a tourniquet are as follows;

- Apply the tourniquet at least 5cm above the wound on the thigh or upper arm. If the injury is below the knee/elbow, apply the tourniquet just above the joint.
- Once applied, tighten the tourniquet until the bleeding begins to reduce and is no longer life threatening.
- Applying a tourniquet is often extremely painful for the casualty. Explain that the pain will usually be temporary and is needed to save their life.
- If bleeding cannot be fully controlled with the tourniquet, consider further application of direct pressure to the wound with a sterile or haemostatic dressing. In some cases, a second, higher tourniquet is necessary.
- Ensure the emergency services have been called on 999/112.
- Note the exact time of application by writing the time on the tourniquet strap or next to the tourniquet on the skin.
- Tourniquets should be fit for purpose and not fabricated by the first aider.

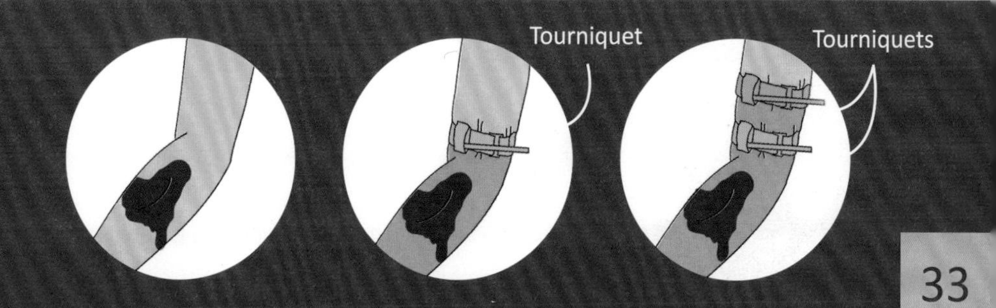

5.4 Embedded Objects

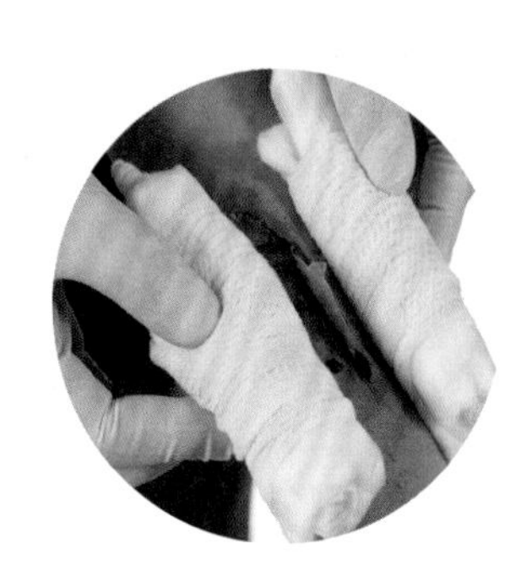

If there is an embedded object in the wound, like a piece of glass, it should not be removed. The 'object' could be stemming the bleeding and removing it could result in internal damage and greater blood loss. Instead, to treat this special type of wound we need to apply direct pressure around the object then build up our dressing, holding the object firmly in place. Casualties with this type of wound must go to hospital to have the object removed.

Splinters are a day to day occurrence in some industries and I'm sure you have had them from time to time.

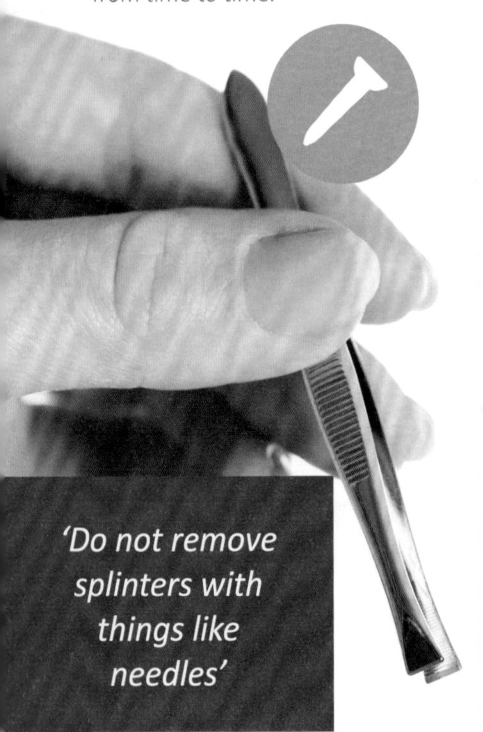

'Do not remove splinters with things like needles'

Treatment (Splinters)

DO NOT remove splinters with things like needles as this may push the splinter deeper and cause more damage.

If possible brush the splinter off with a blunt edge (side of a credit card), your finger or use a pair of tweezers.

Once the splinter is removed, squeeze the wound gently to encourage bleeding as this will help remove any dirt, then clean and dress the wound.

The casualty should consider seeking medical advice about receiving a tetanus injection if they haven't had one recently.

5.5 Nosebleed

One of the most common injuries you may be expected to deal with is a nosebleed. Simple things like a bang to the nose, picking or blowing the nose can lead to the nose bleeding but there may also be more serious causes, such as a **skull fracture** or **high blood pressure**.

Treatment

Sit the casualty down and get them to tilt their head forwards.

Pinch the soft part of the nose for ten minutes. Have the casualty breathe through their mouth.

Have a cloth or bowl readily available for any drips or dribbles.

After ten minutes allow the casualty to stop pinching the nose.

If the bleeding has stopped: Advise the casualty to rest and not to pick or blow their nose for several hours, as this may disturb any blood clots that have formed resulting in the nose bleeding again.

If the bleeding continues: Pinch the soft part of the nose again for a further ten minutes.

If the nosebleed continues for longer than 30 minutes: Send or take the casualty to hospital.

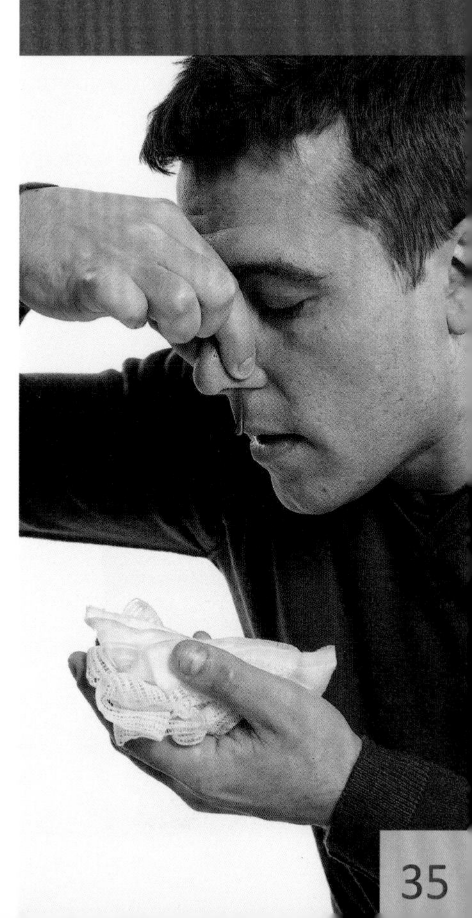

5.6 Eye Injuries

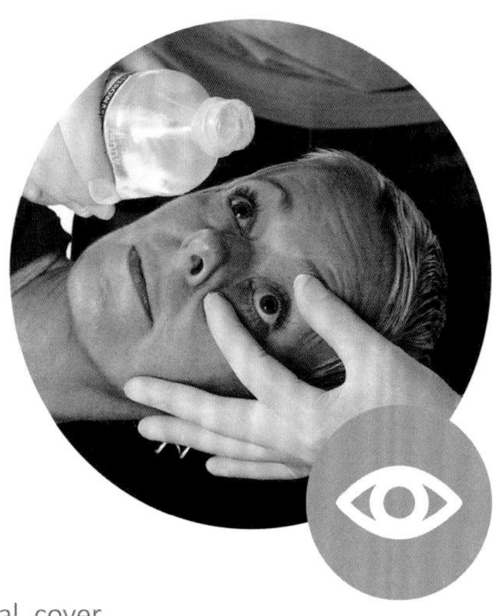

Eye wounds are a concern for a first aider because the risk to a casualty's vision is serious. **DO NOT** attempt to touch or remove anything embedded in the eyeball.

Treatment

Small particles may be washed away using a sterile eye wash or clean running water but you may not be able to see any scratches or damage done to the eye as a result of the injury.

To protect the casualty's eye on route to hospital, cover with a sterile dressing, and secure into position. Then ask the casualty to rest their good eye to prevent movement of the injured eye. You will need to reassure the casualty throughout this treatment.

5.7 Internal Bleeding

'One of the most difficult injuries to recognise as a first aider is internal bleeding'

One of the most difficult injuries to recognise as a first aider is internal bleeding. For a start you can't see it and it manifests itself in different ways.

Recognition

The main signs of internal bleeding you would recognise are (either sign would indicate a serious underlying illness or injury and must be treated as such):

- the casualty going into shock and/or
- bleeding from an orifice.

5.8 Shock

Shock is caused by the failure of the circulatory system. In simple terms that means the vital organs, including the brain and heart, are not getting enough oxygenated blood. This condition is potentially life threatening and requires immediate action to prevent it's onset or to treat it.

Shock can be caused by the loss of bodily fluids through severe bleeding, vomiting, diarrhoea, severe burns or excess sweating. It can also be caused by a dilation of the blood vessels as a result of infection or a spinal cord injury.

Recognition

- Pale, cold and clammy skin
- Sweating
- Rapid, weak pulse
- Rapid, shallow breathing
- Nausea
- Thirst
- Dizziness / light-headedness

'DO NOT allow casualty to eat or drink'

Treatment

- Treat the cause of shock
- Lay the casualty down on the floor
- Elevate and support the legs above the level of the heart
- Loosen clothing, neck, chest and waist
- Keep the casualty warm
- Reassure the casualty
- Call 999/112 and ask for an ambulance
- Continue to monitor casualty's breathing and airway until help arrives
- **DO NOT** allow casualty to eat or drink
- Be prepared to resuscitate

We must advise - Diabetics should follow their diet plan + management techniques - check bloods + take sugar etc. as required.

they can have a sip of water

Bones, Muscle & Joint Injuries

6.1 Head Injuries

Head injuries are a concern for first aiders as they are potentially very serious and could lead to your casualty becoming unresponsive. In this section we are going to cover three different head injuries you may come across, a skull fracture, compression and concussion.

Concussion

Concussion is caused when the casualty's brain is shaken within the skull by a blow or bang to the head. Typically the casualty will lose responsiveness briefly (a minute or so) leading to short term memory loss of the event that caused the injury but then they should make a full recovery.
A note of caution: be aware of potential spinal injury.

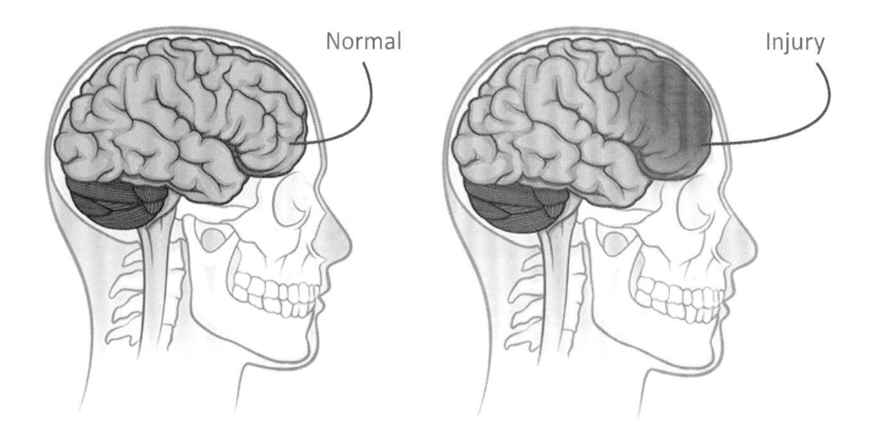

Recognition

- Brief loss of responsiveness
- Nausea, mild headache, dizziness
- Loss of memory

Treatment

- If unresponsive, place in the recovery position
- Call 999/112 and ask for an ambulance
- Monitor airway, breathing and level of response
- If the casualty remains responsive following the blow to their head, monitor vital signs and if their level of response begins to deteriorate after their initial recovery call 999/112 and ask for an ambulance

Skull Fracture

The skull protects the brain and the brain is attached to the spinal cord. As a result, any injury to the skull can affect our central nervous system (CNS). The job of the CNS is to control important body functions like breathing, body temperature and circulation, so any damage caused by an injury to the head can affect these vital functions.

Recognition

- A wound to the skull
- Impaired level of responsiveness
- Blood or clear fluid leaking from the ears and/or nose
- Headache
- Confusion or strange behaviour

Treatment

- Treat any wounds/bleeding or fluid loss as you find them
- Sit the casualty in a comfortable position
- If there is swelling use a cold compress
- Monitor casualty for signs of deterioration
- Call 999/112 and ask for an ambulance
- Be prepared to place the casualty in the recovery position or resuscitate

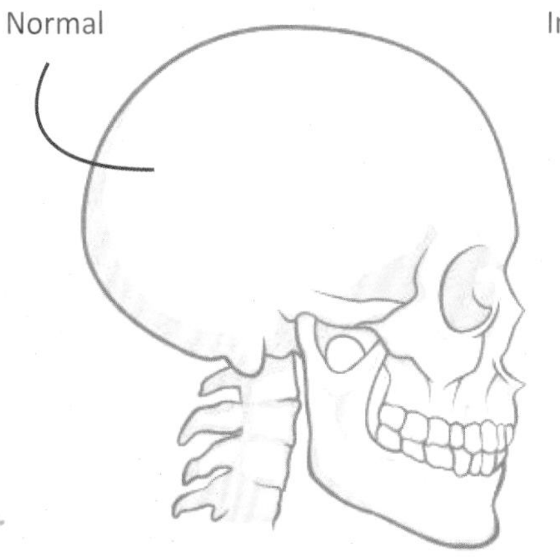

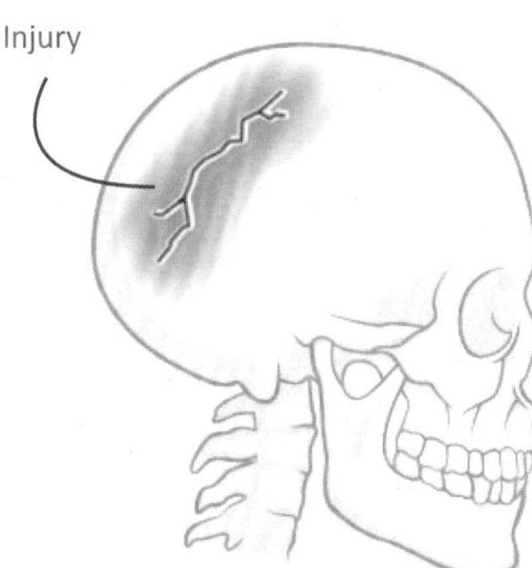

Bones, Muscle & Joint Injuries
Head Injuries

Cerebral Compression

The most serious head injury you may need to deal with is cerebral compression. This is where pressure builds up on the brain within the skull as a result of internal bleeding, swelling of the brain tissue or infection. Compression may occur directly after a blow to the head or it may take several days to develop.

Recognition

- Deteriorating level of response
- Evidence of a head injury
- Intense headache
- Noisy, slow breathing
- Strong, slow pulse
- High temperature
- Unequal pupil size
- Change in personality or behaviour

Treatment

- If the casualty is responsive, lay them down and support their head and shoulders
- Call 999/112 and ask for an ambulance, remember this is a serious medical condition
- If the casualty is unresponsive, manage their airway, but leave in the position they have been found because of the possible risk of a spinal injury
- Be prepared to resuscitate

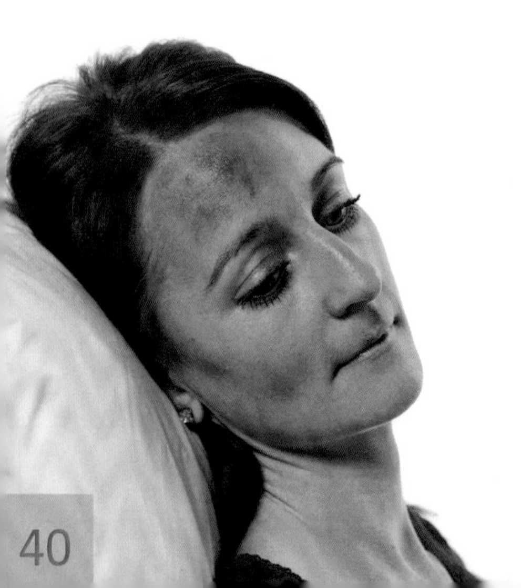

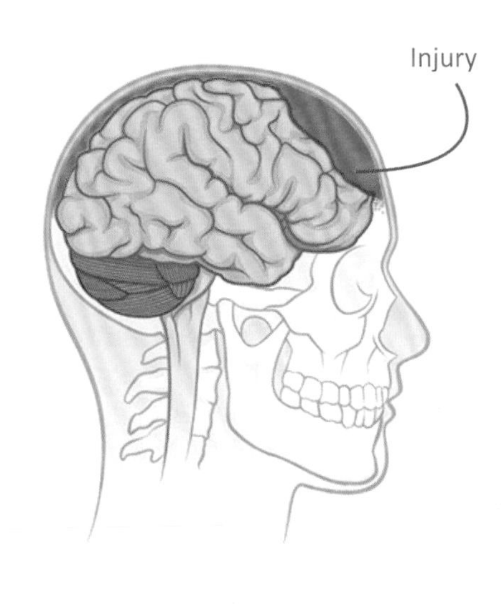

6.2 Spinal Injuries

The spinal column is part of the central nervous system along with the brain. The spine is made up of vertebrae (bones), discs, soft tissues and the spinal cord.

The purpose of the spine is to protect the spinal cord and aid movement. As a first aider it is very important that you are aware of spinal injuries and the possible damage caused. When suspecting a spinal injury you need to take into account the mechanism of the injury, which means how the injury occurred.

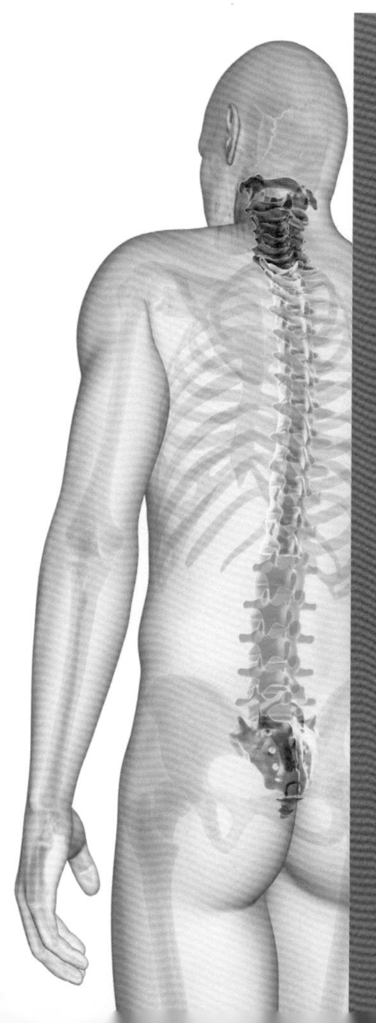

Recognition

Vertebrae or Discs:

- Pain at the site of the injury
- A twist or step in the normal shape of the spine
- Bruising or tenderness at the injury site

Spinal Cord :

- Loss of control of limbs
- Loss of movement
- Breathing difficulty
- Abnormal sensations (tingling, pins & needles, burning)
- Loss of bladder control

Possible Causes

- Falling from height
- Falling from a horse or moving vehicle
- Falling awkwardly
- Collapsed rugby scrum
- Injury to the head or face
- Heavy object falling across the back
- Diving into a shallow swimming pool and hitting the bottom

Bones, Muscle & Joint Injuries

Spinal Injuries

Treatment (Responsive Casualty not in Imminent Danger)

You should not move a casualty with a suspected spinal injury if they are not in imminent danger. Leave the casualty in the position you found them and support the casualty's head and neck. The main aims of treating a casualty with a suspected spinal injury are to:

- Prevent further injury
- Manage the airway
- Call 999/112 for an ambulance

'DO NOT move the casualty unless they are in imminent danger'

Supporting head and neck

- Reassure the casualty and tell them not to move.
- Kneel behind the casualty's head. Place your hands on either side of the casualty's head with your fingers pointing towards the casualty's body.
- **DO NOT** cover their ears, as they need to listen to your instructions and reassurance.
- Supporting the head in this neutral position will align the head, neck and spine and prevent any movement.
- Continue to reassure the casualty, keep them warm, and tell them not to move.
- Continue to do this until medical assistance arrives.

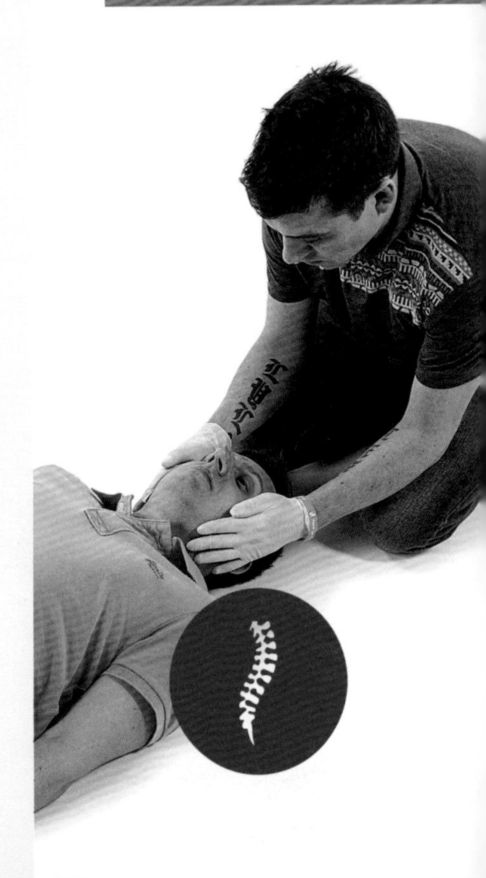

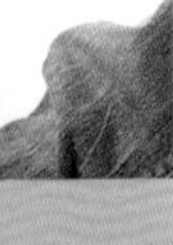

Treatment (Responsive Casualty in Imminent Danger - Log Roll)

You would only move a casualty with a suspected spinal injury if they were in imminent danger. For example vomiting, as this would compromise their airway or danger from fire, flames, traffic, etc. Moving the casualty before the ambulance arrives is a last resort and should ideally be done with enough helpers. The technique for moving the casualty is known as the 'log roll' and can only be attempted if you have help.

Log Roll

Straighten the casualty's limbs. Then when everyone is ready, begin rolling the casualty in one slow, steady, controlled movement. Keep the casualty's head, chest, hips and legs supported at all times maintaining a straight spine.

One helper: Support the head and neck as previous page. Your helper then turns the body as you stabilise the head.

Three or more helpers: Support the neck and head as above. Position your remaining helpers along the length of the casualty's body. Ideally you need three on one side of the body so they can pull the casualty towards them whilst the additional helpers position themselves on the opposite side ready to assist the roll.

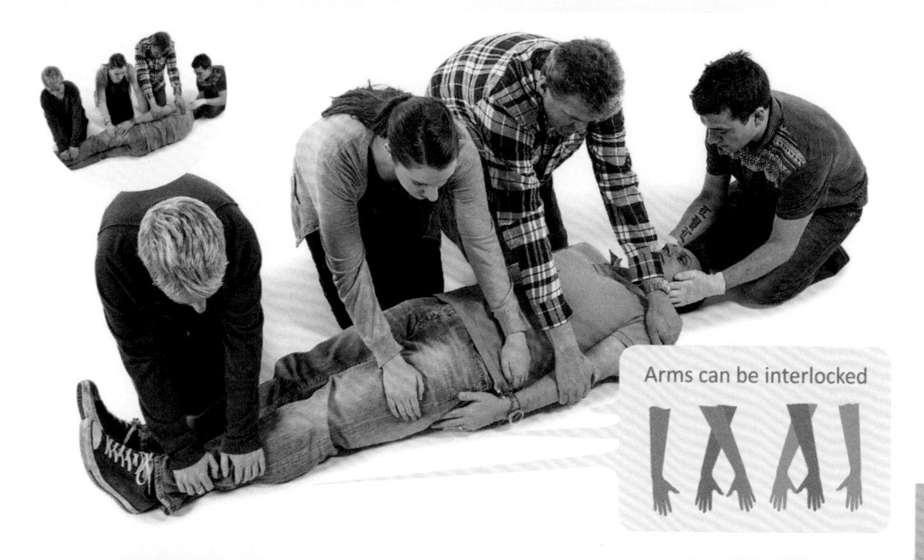

Bones, Muscle & Joint Injuries

Spinal Injuries

Treatment (Unresponsive Casualty - Recovery Position)

As always with an unresponsive casualty we are concerned about managing the casualty's airway and breathing. We also know that we **DO NOT** want to move them unless it is really necessary. So how do we do this?

If you are alone and you have to leave the casualty who is unresponsive and breathing normally, to call for an ambulance, you must place them in the recovery position as this is the only way to manage their airway. Upon returning to your casualty, leave them in the recovery position.

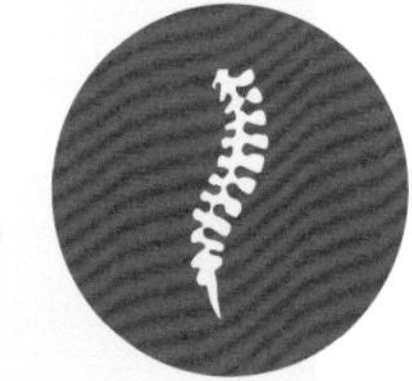

If you have summoned help already for an unresponsive casualty who is breathing normally then you can manage their airway and breathing by performing a simple head tilt, chin lift. Ensuring minimum movement of the casualty. If the casualty stops breathing normally, you will have to begin CPR.

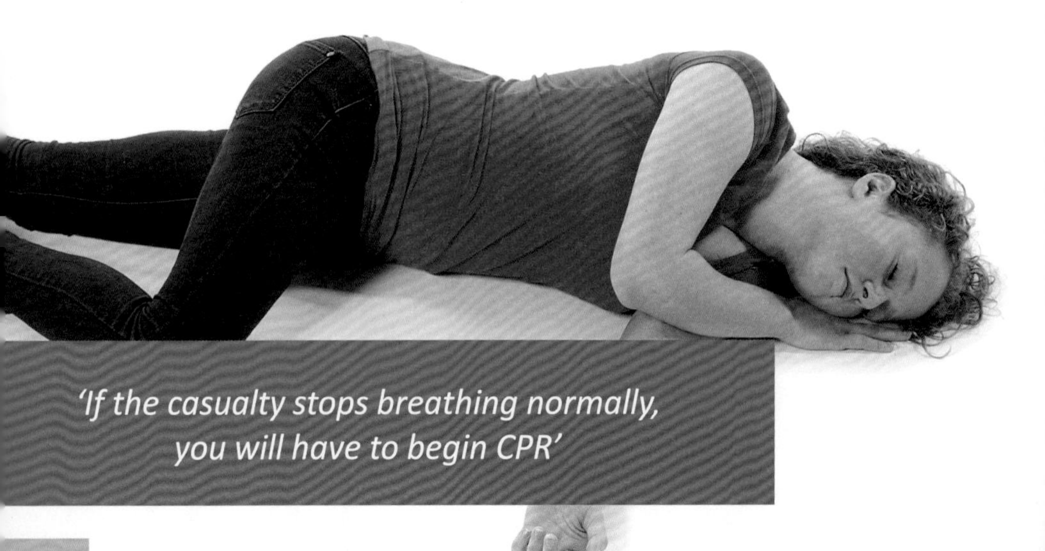

'If the casualty stops breathing normally, you will have to begin CPR'

6.3 Chest Injury

Injuries to the chest can be serious as they can affect the casualty's breathing.

Fractured ribs caused by a blow to the chest can be painful and uncomfortable but if the blow is significant the ribs could cause damage to the lungs, heart or liver causing internal bleeding.

'Injuries to the chest can be serious as they can affect the casualty's breathing'

Recognition

- Pain, swelling and bruising at the site of the injury
- Discomfort and pain when breathing
- Shallow breathing
- Possible signs of hypoxia
- Possible signs of internal bleeding, coughing up of bright red, frothy blood
- You may be able to hear the sound of air being sucked into the chest cavity

Treatment

- Support the casualty into a sitting position leaning towards the injured side
- If the wound is bleeding, control with direct pressure
- Call 999 / 112 and ask for an ambulance
- Monitor the casualty's breathing and level of response until help arrives

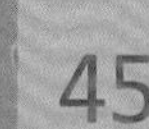

Bones, Muscle & Joint Injuries

6.4 Broken Bones (Fractures)

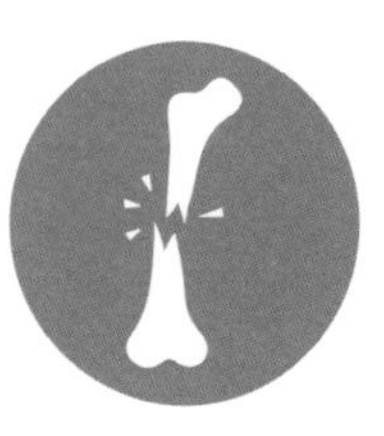

There are 206 bones which make up the human skeleton. The purpose of the skeleton is to protect the vital organs and act as a framework for the soft tissues, joints, muscles, tendons and ligaments. Bones are relatively difficult to break (fracture). Bones break as a result of direct force (being struck by a heavy blow) or by indirect force (a twisting movement).

The resulting broken bone may be classed as closed (where the skin isn't punctured), open (where the broken bone punctures the skin creating a wound) or complicated (where complications have arisen as a result of the fracture, such as trapped blood vessels or nerves).

Recognition

- Pain at the site of the injury
- Irregularity, deformity, swelling, bruising
- Difficulty moving the limb
- Crepitus (grinding of the bone ends where it is broken)

Treatment

- Immobilise and support the injured limb in the most comfortable position for the casualty
- This may or may not include slings and bandages
- Treat or prevent the casualty for shock
- Call 999/112 for an ambulance

6.5 Dislocation

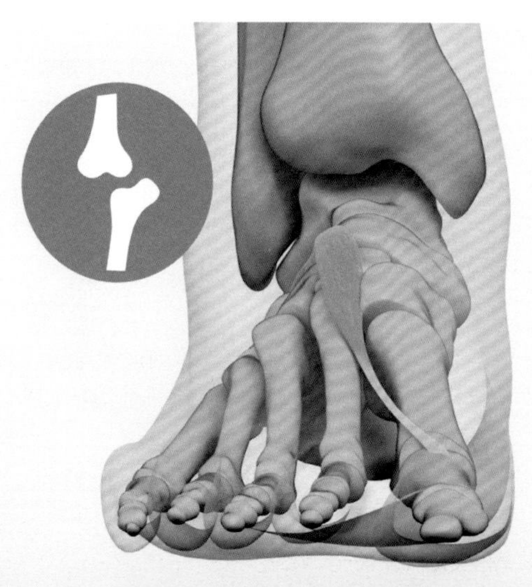

A dislocation occurs when two halves of a joint are separated. Dislocations are incredibly painful as the bone is pulled out of its normal position. Joints can be found in the knee, fingers, vertebrae, shoulder, elbow, hip and jaw. Recognition and treatment are as per broken bones. NO attempt should be made by a first aider to 'pop' the joint back into position!

6.6 Sprains and Strains

Sprains and strains are injuries to the soft tissues. A sprain is a tear of the ligaments around a joint whilst a strain is a tear of the muscles and tendons.

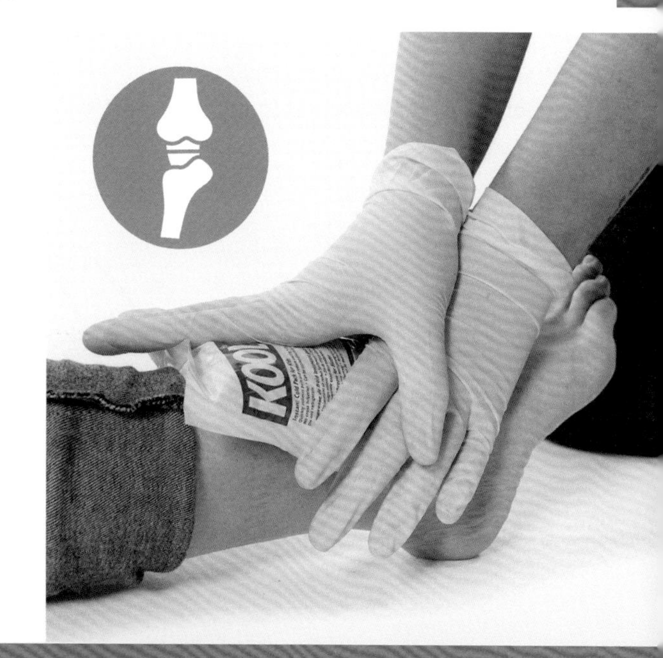

Recognition

- Pain
- Inflammation
- Swelling
- Tenderness
- Inability to move the affected area

Treatment (RICE)

Sprains and strains are treated in the same way by using the 'RICE' method. The aim of this treatment is to reduce swelling and the associated pain as quickly as possible. If you are in any doubt as to the severity of the injury, treat as a fracture and arrange for transportation to a hospital.

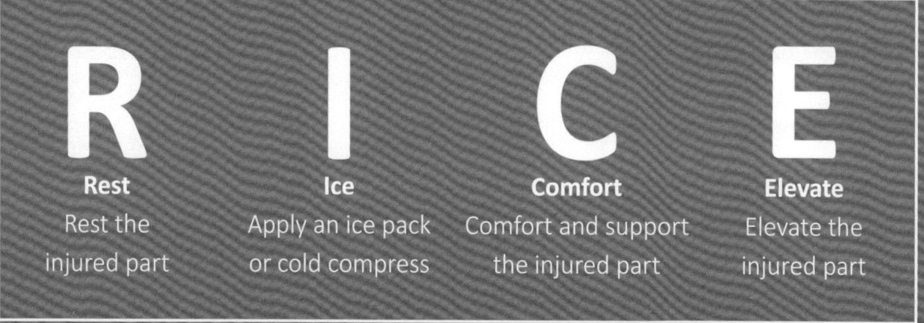

Burns & Scalds

7.1 The Skin

The skin is one of the largest and most important organs in the body. It consists of various layers; the epidermis (outer layer) and the dermis (the inner layer) below which sits a layer of subcutaneous fat.

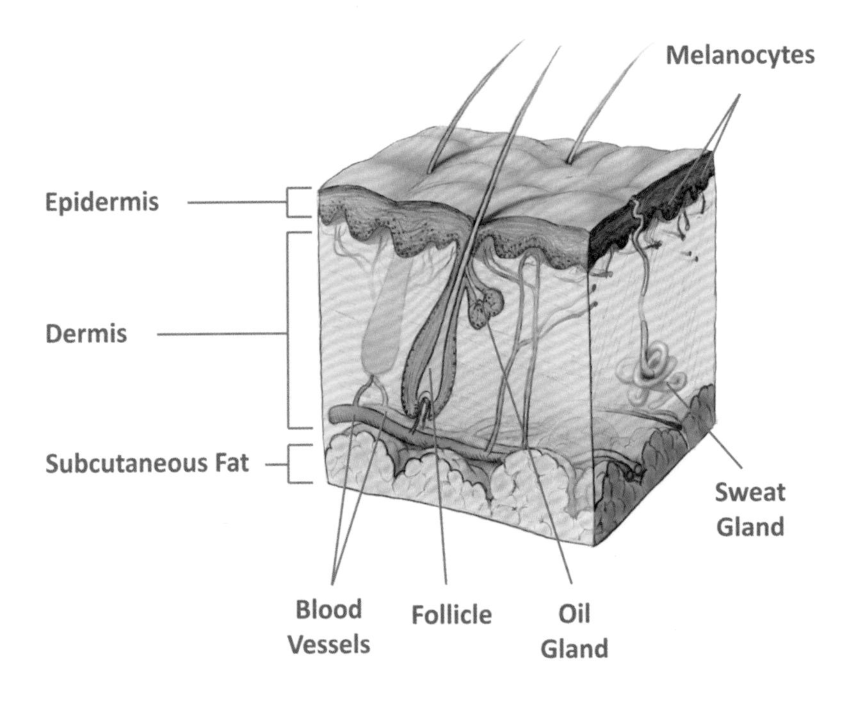

The main purpose of the skin is to help maintain our temperature, retain water and protect the body from injury and infection. Any damage to the skin is painful because of the number of nerve endings.

The skin can be burnt in many ways, all are painful but the major concern with burns is the high risk of infection and the loss of bodily fluids.

'Any damage to the skin is painful because of the number of nerve endings'

7.2 Depth of Burns

A burn is classified by its depth and the damage to the skin.

1. Superficial burn

   This burn affects the outermost layer of skin the epidermis. Superficial burns look red in colour, are tender to the touch and swelling may occur.

2. Partial-thickness burn

   This burn looks and feels similar to a superficial burn but is worse as blisters are present. Partial-thickness burns are usually very painful. **DO NOT** burst blisters as they are helping prevent infection.

3. Full-thickness burn

   This burn affects all the layers of the skin (epidermis and dermis), they may even burn the skin as far down as the layer of subcutaneous fat and muscles. This type of burn may look pale, black, charred and waxy and requires urgent medical attention. Full-thickness burns are usually painless. This is because the nerve endings have been burnt away.

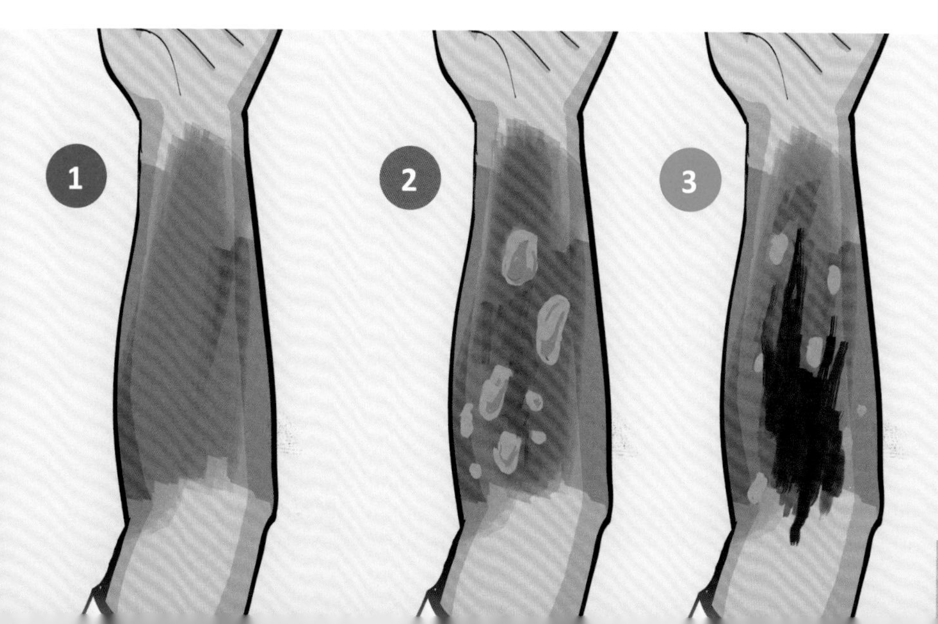

Burns & Scalds

7.3 Types of Burns

Scalds
Steam and hot liquids.

Dry Burn
Friction, flames, and hot surfaces.

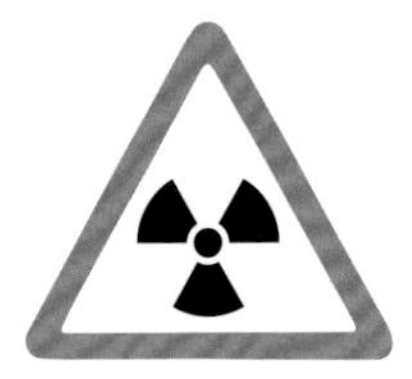

Radiation Burns
Sunburn, sun beds (ultraviolet light) and X-rays.

Electrical Burns*
Domestic appliances (low voltage), overhead power lines (high voltage), and lightning.

Cold Injury
Frozen metal objects, frostbite and freezing vapours.

Chemical Burns*
Domestic chemicals (bleach, oven cleaner, etc.) and industrial chemicals (gases, acids, alkaline).

**Electrical burns:* Be aware that electrical burns may have two burns, an entry and exit point and that the electricity may have caused internal damage as the electricity passed through the body. Electric shocks may also cause the casualty to go into cardiac arrest. Be prepared to resuscitate.

**Chemical burns:* Chemical burns are always serious and will need medical assistance. Treat chemical burns with caution as you do not want to disperse the chemical when flushing with water or get the chemical on yourself. Cool the affected area for a minimum of 20 minutes rather than the usual 10 minutes. Remove any contaminated clothing whilst cooling with water. Refer to COSHH and safety data sheets.

7.4 Treatment for Burns

DO NOT burst blisters.
DO NOT remove clothing that is stuck to the skin.
DO NOT apply any lotions, creams or ointments as this damages the skin and increases the risk of infection.
DO NOT touch the burnt area.

Cool the burn down under cold running water for a minimum of 10 minutes.

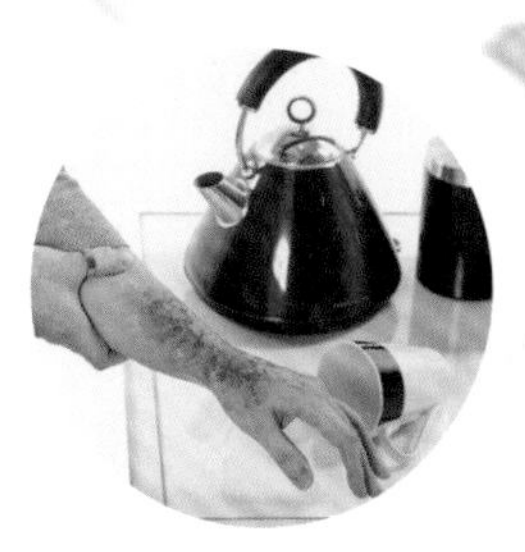

Remove any watches and jewellery (especially rings) before tissues begin to swell.

To protect the burnt area from infection cover with cling film. If none is available use a non fluffy sterile dressing.

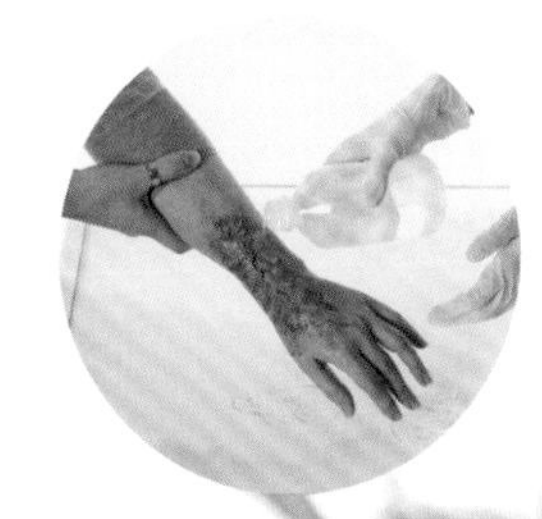

Treat the casualty for shock (or the prevention of it).

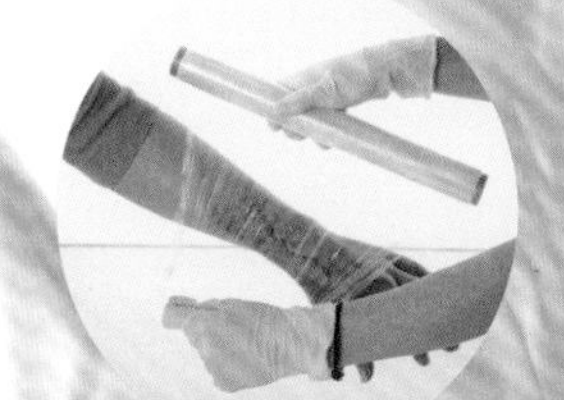

If appropriate call 999/112 for an ambulance.

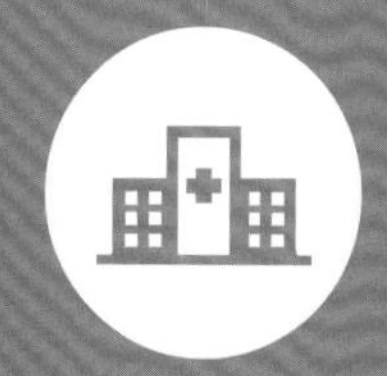

Must be treated in a hospital:

- Burns to children and infants, regardless of the depth.
- All full thickness burns.
- All burns that extend around an arm or leg.
- ALL burns involving the face, genitals, hands or feet.
- All partial thickness burns that are larger than 1% of a casualty's body surface.
- All superficial burns that are larger than 5% of the casualty's body surface.
- Burns that have a mixed depth pattern.

Poisoning

8.1 How Poisons Enter the Body

Poisons enter the body through many routes. They can be swallowed, inhaled through the nose or mouth, injected or absorbed through the skin or splashed (instilled) into the eye. Once they enter the body, poisons can work in many different ways. Some signs and symptoms can be mild, others life threatening, depending on the poison and the quantity that has entered the body. The definition of a poison is any substance taken in sufficient quantity that can cause temporary or permanent damage to the body. Always check the label on the substance a casualty has taken to find out information on how to treat them.

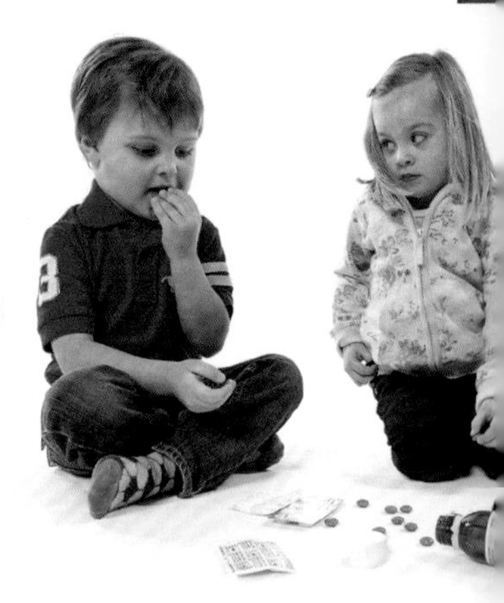

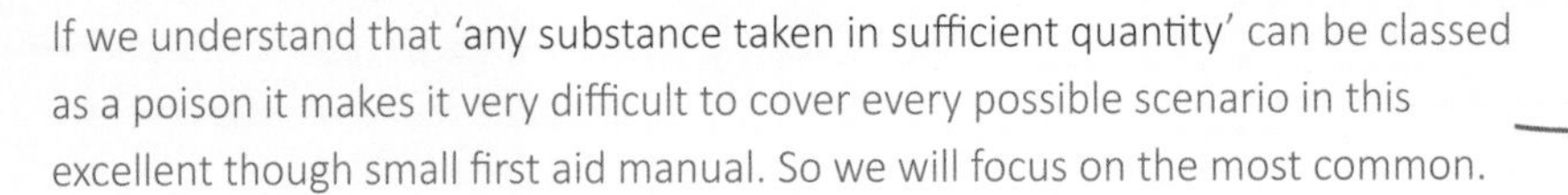

8.2 Types of Poison

If we understand that 'any substance taken in sufficient quantity' can be classed as a poison it makes it very difficult to cover every possible scenario in this excellent though small first aid manual. So we will focus on the most common.

8.3 Sources of Information

Household and industrial chemicals contain clear labels and safety data sheets which display vital information on:

- How to use (e.g. shake well before use)
- How to store (e.g. out of direct sunlight)
- How to dispose of the product
- What protection you require to use the product (e.g. protective gloves required)
- What to do in the event of an emergency (e.g. wash hands and exposed skin after use)

You can receive further information by visiting the NHS websites or contacting the local ambulance service during an emergency. Have the following information to hand so that you receive the best possible advice; what has been taken, how much has been taken and when it was taken.

Injected Poisons

Recognition: Localised pain, swelling and redness around the area of the injection, possible anaphylactic reaction, nausea and vomiting, difficulty in breathing, an impaired level of responsiveness.

Causes: Bites and stings from animals, drugs.

Treatment: For bites and stings, if possible, remove the sting by scraping off; **DO NOT** use tweezers to squeeze the sting as this may add additional poison. If the sting cannot be removed seek medical attention and monitor for signs of anaphylactic shock.

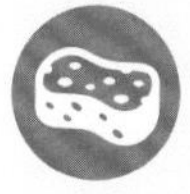

Absorbed Poisons

Recognition: Localised pain, swelling and redness. Rash and itching may develop.

Causes: Household chemicals, Industrial chemicals, plant poisons.

Treatment: Wash the area for 20 minutes if it is a chemical burn/poison and call 999/112 for an ambulance. Be prepared to resuscitate.

Splashed in the Eye (instilled)

Recognition: Pain in and around the eye, the eye will water and the casualty may have difficulty opening or seeing out of the affected eye.

Causes: Chemicals, plant poisons, smoke, toxic fumes.

Treatment: Flush the eye with plenty of water, if it is a chemical do this for 20 minutes, be sure you **DO NOT** allow contaminated water to run into the 'good' eye, dress the eye with a non fluffy dressing and seek immediate medical assistance.

Swallowed Poisons

Recognition: Possible burning sensation around the mouth and throat, abdominal pain, nausea, vomiting, difficulty breathing, seizures and an impaired level of responsiveness.

Causes: Household chemicals, plant poisons, drugs, foods, alcohol.

Treatment: Identify the poison taken, sit casualty down. **DO NOT** induce vomiting, keep the casualty still and call 999/112 for an ambulance. Be prepared to resuscitate (using a face shield or pocket mask).

Inhaled Poisons

Recognition: Difficulty breathing, dizziness, hypoxia, impaired level of responsiveness.

Causes: Smoke, toxic fumes from chemicals, and drugs.

Treatment: Move the casualty into fresh air if it is safe to do so and call 999/112 for an ambulance. Be prepared to resuscitate (using a face shield or pocket mask).

Medical Emergencies

9.1 Anaphylaxis

'Allow the casualty to take their own medication'

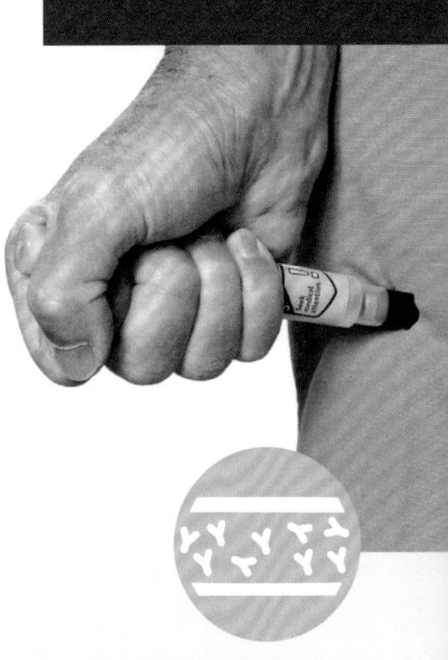

Anaphylactic shock is a life threatening, severe allergic reaction that affects the whole body as the body produces massive amounts of histamine to combat a perceived threat.

The production of histamine dilates the blood vessels leading to a fall in blood pressure and difficulty breathing as the airways begin to constrict. Known sufferers of anaphylaxis will carry their own medication by way of an auto injector of adrenaline (epinephrine).

Anaphylactic shock can be triggered by eating items like shellfish, nuts, medicines and dairy products or from coming into contact with chemicals, animals and insects (i.e. wasp or bee stings).

Recognition

- Swelling of hands and feet
- Swelling of face, neck, mouth and tongue
- Difficulty in breathing
- Anxiety and distress
- Pale or flushed skin
- Impaired level of responsiveness
- Signs and symptoms of shock
- Pain, swelling and redness around the area of the contact

Treatment

- Call 999/112 for an ambulance
- Allow the casualty to sit in a position which aids their breathing
- Allow the casualty to take their own medication
- If they are unable to take their own medication you may use the auto injector to administer the medication for them (this procedure may be repeated at 5-15 minute intervals if no improvement or the symptoms return)
- Be prepared to treat for the onset of shock
- Be prepared to resuscitate

9.2 Angina

Angina pectoris is the narrowing of the coronary arteries. If a sufferer of angina places additional stress on the heart through exertion then the heart cannot supply itself with sufficient blood to function properly. This results in an angina attack which the sufferer can treat by resting and taking their own medication.

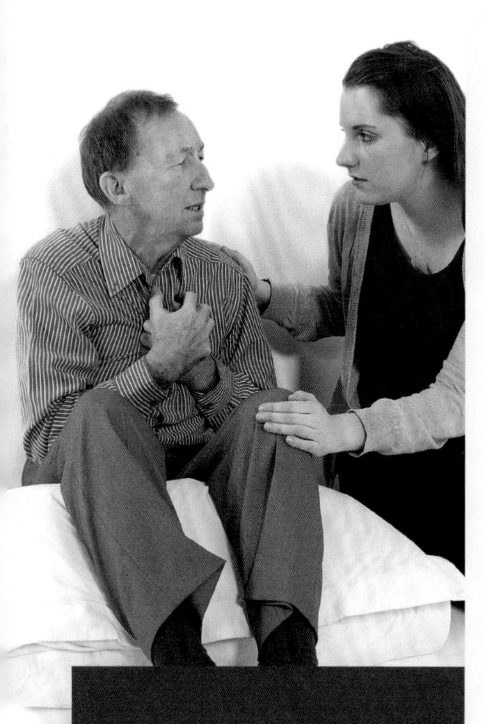

'An angina attack which the sufferer can treat by resting and taking their own medication'

Recognition

- Vice like, crushing chest pain which may radiate down the arm(s) or up to the jaw
- Rapid breathing
- Shortness of breath
- Fear and anxiety
- Pale, cold and clammy skin

Treatment

- Pain will ease with rest
- Sit the casualty down on the floor and bend and support the knees
- Allow the casualty to take their own medication, assist them to do so if necessary
- If the pain does not ease with rest, treat as a heart attack
- Call 999/112 and ask for an ambulance
- Be prepared to resuscitate

Medical Emergencies

9.3 Heart Attack

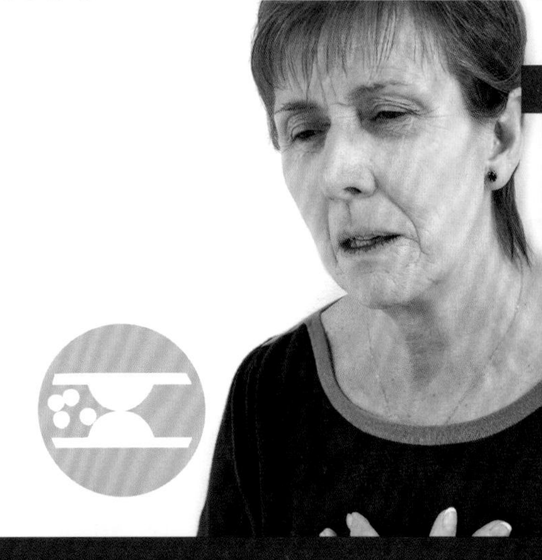

It is estimated that someone has a heart attack in the UK every two minutes. That's about 275,000 people a year of which 120,000 will be fatal.

A heart attack (also known as a Myocardial Infarction) is caused by a blockage (clot) in the coronary arteries. As a result of this blockage, part of the heart muscle is deprived of blood and oxygen. The muscle begins to die and the heart cannot function properly. Ultimately the heart will stop beating and the sufferer will die. Clearly time is an issue here as a heart attack is a life threatening medical emergency.

'Someone has a heart attack in the UK every two minutes'

Recognition

- Vice like, crushing chest pain which may radiate down the arm(s) or up to the jaw
- Rapid breathing
- Shortness of breath
- Rapid or irregular pulse
- Fear and anxiety
- Impending sense of doom
- Pale, cold and clammy skin, 'ashen' in colour, blueness around the lips
- Collapse without warning

Treatment

- Unlike angina the pain will NOT ease with rest
- Sit the casualty down on the floor and bend and support the knees
- Call 999/112 and ask for ambulance, mention you suspect a heart attack
- Assist the casualty to take 300mg of aspirin (ensure they are not allergic first) advise them to chew it slowly
- Allow the casualty to take their own angina medication, assist them to do so if necessary
- Ensure the casualty rests and remains calm
- Locate AED and be prepared to resuscitate in the event that conditions worsen

9.4 Asthma

Asthma is a condition that affects the airways. During an Asthma attack the muscles around the walls of the airways tighten, become narrower and go into spasm, making breathing very difficult for the sufferer.

An Asthma sufferer will be prescribed several different types of medication. A preventer inhaler has a brown, red or orange cap and is of little use during an acute attack. A reliever inhaler is usually coloured blue and contains a drug which will treat an acute attack.

Recognition

- Difficulty in breathing, especially breathing out
- Wheezy breathing
- Difficulty in speaking
- Coughing
- Signs of anxiety and distress
- Hypoxia and cyanosis

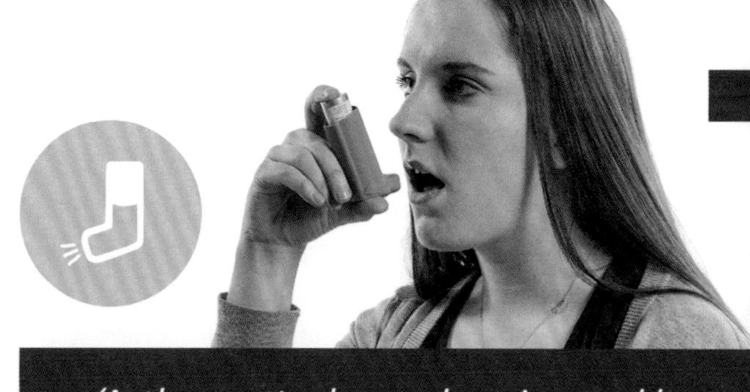

'Asthma attacks can be triggered by allergies, stress, exercise, colds, and changes in temperature'

Treatment

- Reassure them and ask them to breathe slowly and deeply which will help them control their breathing.
- Help them use their reliever inhaler straight away. This should relieve the attack.
- Next, sit them down in a comfortable position.
- If it doesn't get better within a few minutes, it may be a severe attack. Get them to take one or two puffs of their inhaler every two minutes, until they've had 10 puffs.
- If the attack is severe and they are getting worse or becoming exhausted, or if this is their first attack, then call 999/112 for an ambulance.
- Help them to keep using their inhaler if they need to.
- If they lose responsiveness at any point, open their airway, check their breathing and prepare to treat someone who's become unresponsive.

9.5 Epilepsy & Seizures

A seizure is an electrical disturbance in the brain, also known as a fit or convulsion. Seizures can be brought on by many things, an injury to the head, lack of oxygen to the brain, poisoning, strokes or an increase in body temperature. A person with epilepsy suffers from recurrent seizures. Be suspicious of cardiac arrest in any casualty presenting with seizures and carefully assess whether the victim is breathing normally.

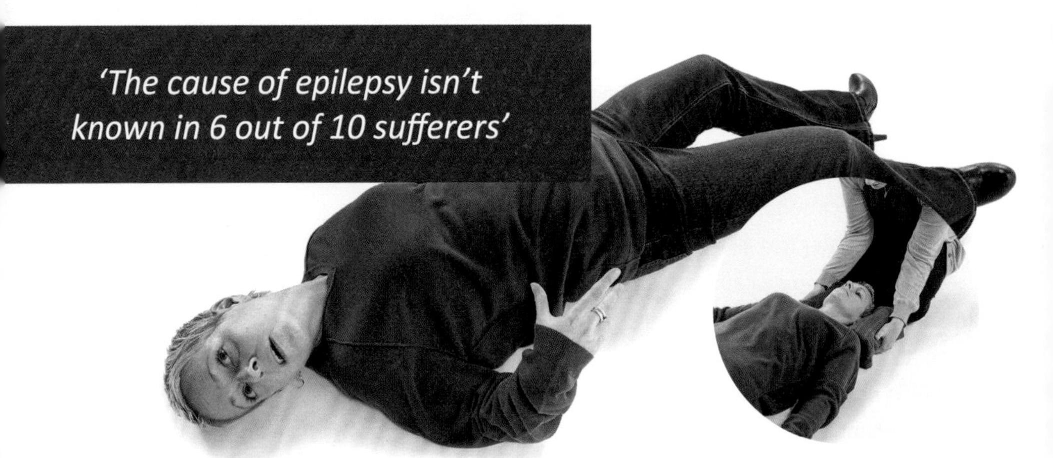

Absence Seizures

Often referred to as a minor or petit mal seizure, sufferers appear to have 'switched off' from their surroundings. This type of seizure may only last a few seconds.

Recognition

- Brief loss of responsiveness
- Distant look on the casualty's face maybe staring blankly
- Twitching of the face, eyes or limbs
- Lip smacking and/or plucking at clothing

Treatment

- Assist the casualty to sit in a quiet place
- Calm and reassure the casualty
- Allow the casualty to recover in their own time
- Be suspicious of cardiac arrest and continue to check for normal breathing

Major Epileptic Seizure

Major epileptic seizures also referred to as grand mal seizures go through two clear phases known as tonic and clonic. These phases are followed by a period of recovery.

Recognition

1. Tonic Phase
   - Casualty loses responsiveness and falls to the ground
   - Rigid arching of the back and the casualty becomes stiff
   - Breathing becomes difficult and you may see signs of cyanosis
   - The phase can last as long as 30 seconds
2. Clonic Phase
   - Casualty begins to convulse/jerk violently
   - Possible loss of bladder or bowel control
3. Recovery
   - The casualty's body now relaxes
   - Normal breathing resumes
   - Casualty remains unresponsive and this may last several minutes

Treatment

- Ensure the area around the casualty is free from danger, so they don't hurt themselves during the seizure
- Cushion and protect the casualty's head but **DO NOT** hold in position
- **DO NOT** place anything in the casualty's mouth or restrain them
- Record the length of the seizure
- Stay with the casualty until their recovery is complete
- Reassure the casualty
- Be suspicious of cardiac arrest and continue to check for normal breathing

Call 999/112 if:

- It is the casualty's first seizure.
- The seizure lasts more than 5 minutes.
- The casualty suffers repeated seizures without regaining responsiveness.
- The casualty becomes injured during the seizure.
- The casualty is unresponsive for longer than 10 minutes.

Medical Emergencies

9.6 Fainting

When somebody faints it's because they have insufficient oxygenated blood reaching their brain. There are many reasons why this could happen: Lack of food, pregnancy, exhaustion, stress, fear or a lack of physical activity which results in the blood pooling in the legs.

Recognition

- Casualty may feel dizzy, lightheaded or nauseous
- Casualty may have no signs or symptoms, they may just fall to the ground
- Brief loss of responsiveness
- Pale, cold and clammy skin
- Have a slow pulse

Treatment

Someone feeling faint:

- Ask the casualty to lie down on the floor, raise their legs higher than their head and support in position
- This will improve the blood flow to their brain
- Expect the casualty to recover quickly

Someone who has fainted:

- If the casualty does not recover in two minutes, place them in the recovery position
- Monitor their airway and breathing
- Call 999/112 for an ambulance
- Be prepared to resuscitate

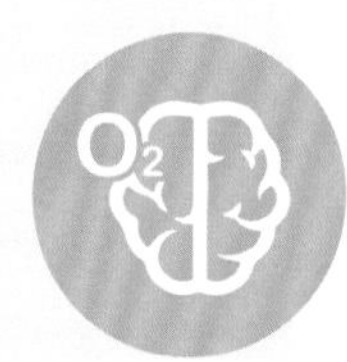

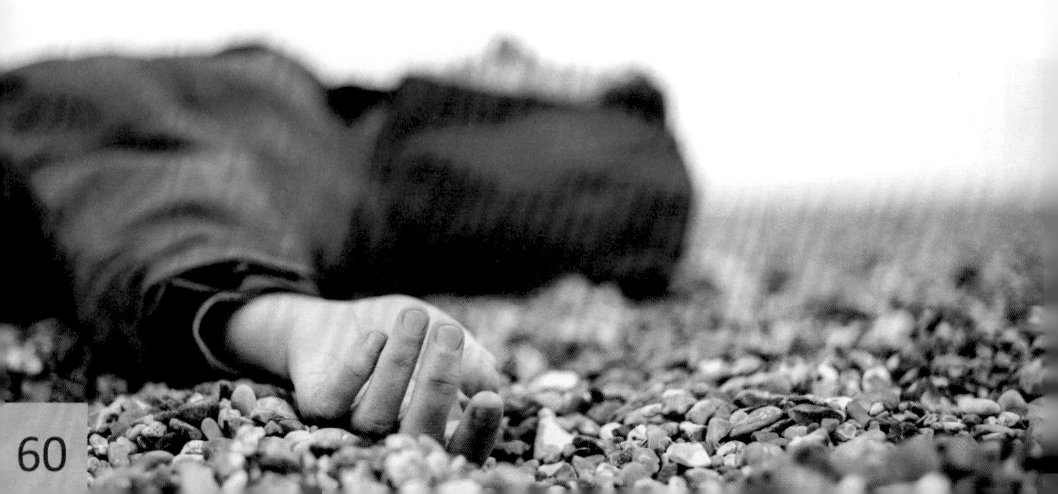

9.7 Stroke

Around 150,000 people a year suffer from a Stroke in the UK, that's one every five minutes! Strokes can happen to anyone, anytime but the majority of Strokes occur to people over 65 years of age. Think of a Stroke as a brain attack that occurs when part of the blood supply to the brain is cut off causing an area of the brain to be damaged or die. Clearly this is a serious condition that requires urgent medical attention. Time is ticking away so you must act FAST. FAST is the recommended guide you should use for a casualty suspected of having a stroke.

Recognition

- Dizziness and confusion
- Sudden severe headache
- Sudden problems with vision, in one or both eyes
- Sudden lack of co-ordination or mobility

Treatment

- Perform the FAST test
- If the casualty fails the test call 999/112 immediately explaining you suspect a stroke
- Allow the casualty to adopt a comfortable position with their head and shoulders raised if conscious
- Reassure and monitor the casualty
- If the casualty becomes unresponsive, place in the recovery position, monitor their airway and breathing
- Call 999/112 for an ambulance
- Be prepared to resuscitate

F – Facial Weakness: Can the casualty smile? Has their eye or mouth drooped?

A – Arm Weakness: Can the person raise BOTH arms?

S – Speech Problems: Can the person speak properly and understand what you say?

T – Time: Time to call 999/112 for anyone you suspect of having a stroke.

9.8 Diabetes

The pancreas is an organ in the body that produces insulin. Our body uses insulin to regulate our blood sugar levels. A person whose body cannot produce sufficient insulin suffers from a medical condition known as diabetes mellitus.

There are two types of Diabetes:

- Type 1 diabetic. The body produces little or no insulin so the sufferer must inject themselves regularly with insulin to control their blood sugar levels.
- Type 2 diabetic. The body produces some insulin, but not enough or it cannot use what it does produce properly.

> *'Hyperglycaemia is a serious medical condition that first aiders can only recognise not treat'*

Hyperglycaemia

This condition is caused by low levels of insulin and high levels of sugar.

Recognition

- Dry, warm skin
- Rapid breathing
- Rapid, weak pulse
- Fruity, sweet smelling breath
- Casualty will be thirsty

Treatment

- Call 999/112 for an ambulance
- Hyperglycaemia is a serious medical condition that first aiders can only recognise not treat
- Be prepared for your casualty to go unresponsive (place in the recovery position)
- Monitor airway and breathing

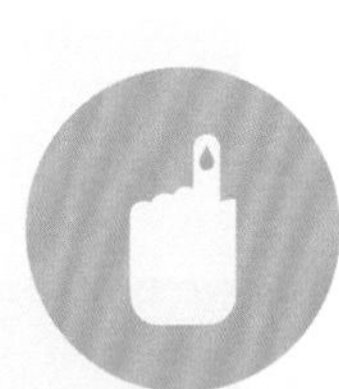

Hypoglycaemia

This condition is caused by high levels of insulin and low levels of sugar.

Recognition

- Pale, cold and clammy skin
- Normal breathing
- Rapid pulse
- Normal smelling breath
- Casualty may suffer from confusion and a change in behaviour (often mistaken for drunkenness)
- Casualty will deteriorate rapidly if treatment not received

Treatment

- Sit the casualty down
- Allow the casualty to take 15-20g of glucose (tablets or gel), if none available give the casualty a sugary drink
- Casualty should respond quickly to the sugar, if they do not call 999/112
- Be prepared for your casualty to go unresponsive (place in the recovery position)
- Monitor airway and breathing

'The casualty may suffer from confusion and a change in behaviour (often mistaken for drunkenness)'

Notes

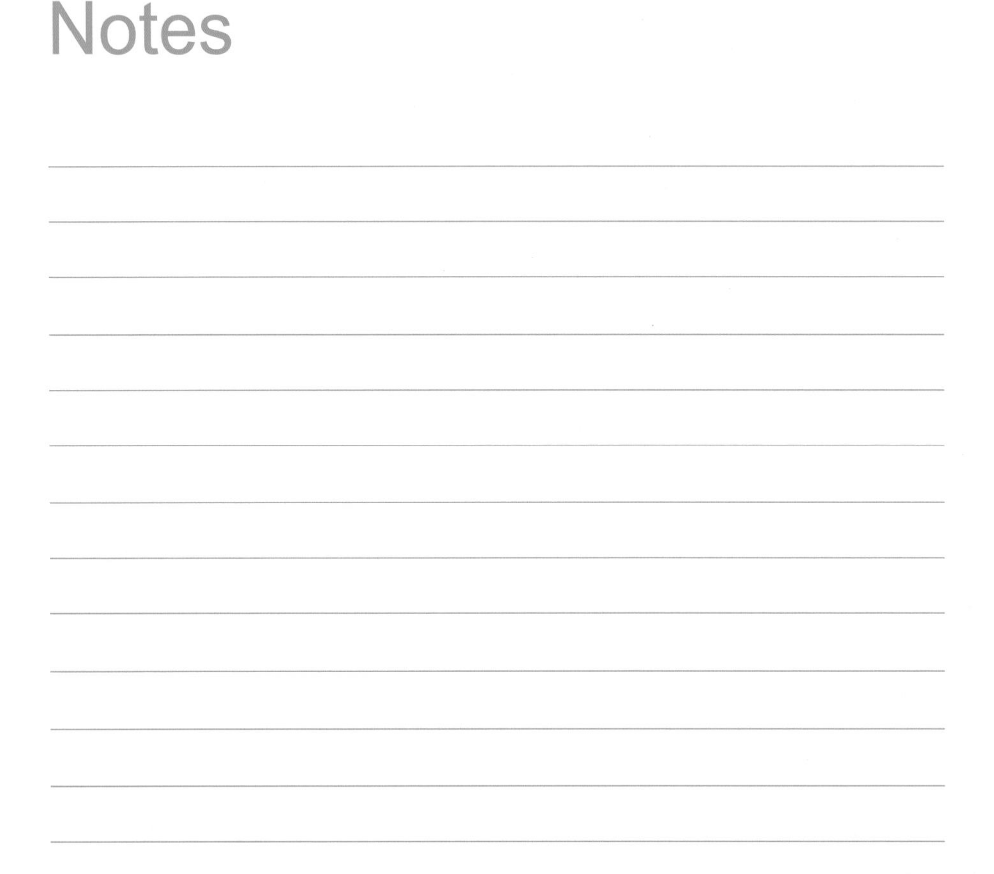

First paperback edition printed 2013 in the United Kingdom.
A catalogue record for this book is available from the British Library. ISBN 978-0-9576376-0-3

Published by Training Qualifications UK Limited. For more copies of this book, please email customerservice@tquk.org.

Tel 0333 358 3344 www.tquk.org

Special Thanks
To everyone involved in making this book possible, especially the willing volunteers who were happy to have their photographs taken along with proof reading and technical support from our Medical Director Frank Cross, Dr Brian Hope and First Aid Advisory Panel.
Finally thanks to Tony West our great photographer and Blanca Martinez Valiente for the fabulous design of the manual.